CONTENTS

CHAPTER 1

Introduction
(the boring bit)

"Life is tough enough without having someone
kick you from the inside." – Rita Rudner

Whatever stage in your pregnancy and childbirth Journey you are at, this is a valuable guide to using simple and effective techniques to build calm and clarity into your pregnancy and child birth experience and to pave the way ahead for your transition into motherhood. Building a deep sense of calm, confidence and a sense of control, centred and Empowered on your journey to and through Motherhood.
Victoria is an Award Winning Personal Empowerment Expert with 21 years experience having qualified in Hypnotherapy specifically for child birth in 2012 ahead of the birth of her son. Victoria has a fascinating insightful dynamic which she is renowned for making the most complex of ideas appear very simple.
Alongside powerful mindset techniques and inspiring motivational perspectives, birthing babies contains fascinating insights into your mind and your body. Its essence and form, and how it is perfectly designed through its evolution, to birth baby with greater ease than you may have foreseen. So you can enjoy the journey you and baby will take together.

Old age wisdom combined with new and dynamic aspects to provide you with a uplifting and enlivening guide to Making child birth more easy, more comfortable and something to enjoy rather than endure.

The recent increase in celebrity and royalty making Hypnotherapy for childbirth more prominent, somehow however right or wrong seems to make it more acceptable.
But it has been around for centuries.
Birthing babies has one simple aim, to make Hypnotherapy for child birth as empowering as possible, simple as possible, as accessible as possible in the modern day. For the woman who is everything.
This simple Guide to a Positively Empowered Birth brings revelatory insights which give the reader the knowledge and power to birth their baby with confidence and create a life beyond birth that is synonymous with the greatest vision they have for their life, beyond birth.
It is more than hypnobirthing you are establishing a new way of living, by restructuring your beliefs as to what is possible as you move forward into parenthood. A new way of making the life you experience forward the life you are choosing, beginning with birth.
On some level, we all want the best for our children we all aspire to be the best parents we can be. We all have aspirations for our lives as parents moving forward and for our children so this is the HOW to set about the ripple in your mind, the ripple in your life that is going to make that happen.
Listen, read, learn, change and then allow the unfolding of life allow the unfolding of you and unfolding of life beyond birth.
The unfolding of a birth where you are calm confident and in control where you are present and one with your body and baby.

It begins

You are pregnant. You might be celebrating or in a place of overwhelm, but it's real. It's happening. And it is ok, even if it does not feel like it.

There is few words that can encapsulate the feeling of pregnancy for the first time as every ones journey is different and every one journey, Is unique.

And that is ok.

The journey can be defined by something more though.

The journey can be defined by your choice to explore the possibilities of a natural birth, or a birth where you are without fear. A birth where you are at one with yourself and at one with baby. A connected birth.

This book will take you through the insights and experience of Doctors and theorists and bring approaches to you that will provide the support the sustenance and the emotional direction to birth baby without fear, to build calm confidence so you are in control in your childbirth experience and with hope allow the wisdom you gain to ripple out into your life.

You can make your birthing journey an empowered one. Not the huge overwhelming power, but the silent inner stance that is educated refined and beautiful. That is power embodied within you as a woman who can birth her baby with confidence.

The natural enhancements. For you as a woman to precede and to predict your life moving forwards by including, and evolving education of the other facts of childbirth. The untold truths that make you more empowered than you could know.

The word empowered is overused now so much it's a branding tool that has been milked of its sentiment of truth. In essence it is within you in its finest form and comes from a silent intention and a silent promise to intend and determine your pregnancy and birthing journey to intend a calm composure and to intend that you know all of the facts and you can enjoy the journey of the evolution moving forward. That is to predict your birthing journey will be one with you and your

intention and one that pervades all challenges. Building a sense of confidence that consumes you when you need it most and believing that the strength within to birth a baby can resonate and resound through all of your life. As the ability to confidently and calmly navigate all challenges overcome with the ability to control and calm your mind, your energy and body into alignment, bringing forth a definite ability to birth your baby with confidence and ease. Birthing babies is about birthing mothers who can, do more than birth, because they birthed. What you learn here will expand into all areas of your life so you can literally change the course of your life for the better through absorbing what you read.

And allowing it to resonate and resound through your life,

encouraging a path that changes the alignment and brings you confidence providing you with solutions, confidence in every aspect of your life moving forward. It brings them through your life as simple stepping stones with which you can easily navigate with a sense of calm composure and grace.

Your pregnancy journey is unique, there are obvious commonalities and likenesses between women, but your body is your own, your vision is your own and your birth is your birth, your babies birth is your birth story as yet unwritten and so to be defined by you. The birth plan is one thing, but your choice to determine how you feel and experience birth is different. You can control the logistics to some extent but you can more effectively control the way you determine your experience inside and that is what is most important.

Birthing babies is a contemporary, empowering and upbeat, guide to birthing your baby with hypnotherapy, but it is more. More than just a book and a series of audio tracks. It's a journey in and of itself and will represent a commitment to you. To change something and to be something that makes your life good.

Bringing the most up to date personal empowerment evolutions and the leading insights in Hypnosis for child birth together to accompany you and guide you on your journey into motherhood. It's an educational journey, aimed to build strengths so you are qualified capable and strong. To define your path as you choose. Designed and authored by World Class Multi Award Winning Personal Empowerment Expert Victoria Whitney.

In person she has a wealth and calm essence. In addition to her wealth of experience the vibrancy and energy she has are unique. The way she works is mysterious but when you look backward in 6 months time you will notice that you have changed and there is something very definite and effortless about that. This is one of the great strengths to working with Victoria.

About Victoria, (yawn...We are here to read about birthing babies so this is brief)

Victoria Whitney LLBhons is an Award Winning Personal Empowerment Expert with 24 years experience having qualified as an Instructor of Hypnotherapy in 2008 and In

Hypnotherapy for Childbirth specifically for child birth in 2012 ahead of the birth of her son. Using Hypnotherapy and learning personal development tools since age 16. Victoria has a fascinating insightful dynamic which she is renowned for making the most complex of ideas appear very simple.

Alongside powerful mind set techniques and inspiring motivational perspectives, birthing babies contains fascinating insights into your physical body it's makeup and its evolution. Everything that you CAN do, You can do, that will influence your life very subtly, but potently.

Pregnancy is a time to nourish yourself as well as baby, even if you don't think you have time. You have a spare 30 minutes here and a spare 30 minutes there. You can find the time. If you look for it. We all have 24 hour days, some people just manage to fit more in. But when you choose to take 10, twenty minutes for purpose it can literally change your life.

The journey you and baby will take together will have highs and lows. There will be moments when you doubt there will be moments of immense joy. Hypnotherapy for child birth has increased in popularity in recent years, the path of celebrity and royalty making Hypnotherapy for childbirth prominent and accessible as possible today, and somehow, right or wrong acceptable.

Working through

1. Introduction - (The boring bit)

2. " Do You want to dance like a chicken." Hypnotherapy Explained.

3. Your body

4. Turning fears into faith

5. Labour

6. Positive affirmations for childbirth

7. "It's all about Positioning baby "

8. Postpartum promise. Beyond birth designing the life you love.

Working through inspiring and identifiable insights to lead you on your road into and through motherhood and introduce you to the ability to confidently navigate the path through planning, pregnancy birth and beyond. Beyond birth you have a future. This book will guide you to establishing the pathways of you real intent for your life. That is the final chapter. It will guide you to lay solid and beautiful foundations for your life. Beyond birth into motherhood.

Even if you aren't pregnant or planning a pregnancy, you may be a midwife or a partner, birth partner of someone who is pregnant. This is the perfect time to envision, learn. Everything you read here will have some resonance, and effect some good change. As you read through the next chapters that will become a new truth for you in some way and you will begin to appreciate the shift in resonance in areas of your life. Especially Your experience of Childbirth.

To define the next steps for life and your pregnancy. From the moment you see the double line on the test strip you know. Everything changes, you feel it... you felt it. You know it. I don't know what you call it but everyone has it. Universally we have the change, the shift. The world turns in an instant and a million thoughts flash through your mind. Either way it turns. However many tests you choose to take. It's real. Life is changed. Celebration, confusion, however it is the feels are real. Feel them. Life is going to change.

And that is Good!

Here is your guide to bring great things into your pregnancy journey, to every day celebrate your body. To merge that energy into intention, whatever you don't know yet can be chosen or learned so for now you can ENJOY.. It's all about education and to embrace the void. Fill it with great things, love, knowledge and all the things you could possibly hope for.

It's natural for a million thoughts to rush through your mind, "How will I ...." " How am I going to .... " The doubts... BOOOOO.

At about this time you will require branded on your consciousness the beliefs.

You are enough.

You can do it.

And it will be ok.

No Matter what

Even when you don't know how.

One day at a time.

How to use this book. Take an open mind and absorb what you choose. What is right for you will naturally permeate your life.

The journey will draw on you in ways you can not even imagine but when you are at the point where you need it you will always have everything you need inside to do the thing that you thought you couldn't do.

Life is going to change in some of the most beautiful and challenging ways. The secret is right here, you are now directing that change. That is the difference. It's true that life will never be the same again and that's a good thing. Whether planned and expected, or unplanned and unexpected. You're reading because you're choosing your path for birthing baby and motherhood with intention.

You have a whole lifetime ahead of you. And that is an opportunity which should never daunt you.

It's totally possible to make sure from the very first thought that it is in alignment with the real vision you have for yourself as a mother or a father and as a women or man.

And that is a gentle process of simply being aware.

Honestly I believe and know that everyone can be empowered to have the life they envisioned, the opportunities experiences, for themselves and their family, all it takes is deliberation and intention. Anyone can (including me) You intend you determine your intentions by moving and being with deliberation. And that kind of unwavering faith. The one that builds when you read books, and learn new ways.

Many women at this time are dawning a new consciousness of determination of natural birth without intervention or asserting the scope of the mind body connection and the bond between mind and body that has always existed. To use it to recognise it.

We are all for medical intervention in childbirth, when it is necessary, but were more for the women to handle the prospect of it in a way that they know they are enough. It does not diminish them in any way, the quality of the mother you become or your worth as a woman is not defined by the success of your birth plan. But that you are aware that you have everything you need inside to do everything you want to do. Everything, even the really really aweful things are overcomable.

So much of our lives people feel determined by others, by circumstances, by the world, by things that are outer to our control. But you realise sometime within sometime in life, preferably now that the most control you have is here in the now.

Pregnancy is the most important time to deliberate the internal interaction you have within. It's a time when most of the natural drains, and impurities are cast aside such as alcohol, caffeine, the crutches. You already go through a phase cleansing like dietary alchemy. Only putting in your body what is good for you and baby. Nourishing your body with foods that are less toxic. Whether it's because you are told to or not it is the best time to also re-engineer the thoughts you have and the intention you have forward, because this is the time when you are most powerful. This is the time.

So to continue to pursue the knowledge and education which enables you to birth your baby into the life you desire. To birth baby with confidence. Birth baby with love. And birth yourself into a phenomenal mother with love and assertion. This is the time. This may sound like something you are already doing but this is another depth.

You can absorb new ideas, explore different ways different concepts right here right now and each and every one will shift something to support you. As you work through this text, you will be reminded to your strengths. There is abundant new knowledge, mostly this is a reminder. Building faith, trust, between your mind and body.

It will at the most basic level shift some fears, educate you in some details you had previously not known which will bring value to you at some time in some place in some space in the future without doubt. And when they do you will remember where they came from, as you allow your self to unfold and enjoy and absorb birthing babies you will find more new possibilities ideas and with intention enjoy the path.

Many women want a natural birth without intervention. For whatever reason, and now you can learn the simple way of the how to do that. You have the scope of the mind body connections and the bond between mind and body that has always existed coherently forever. To use this connection, harness it learn it and evolve into and through it to birth baby calmly and confidently.

Pregnancy and child birth is one of the biggest changes your body can entail. When you think from conception to birth the evolution of your body babies body and then the evolution of the postpartum promise it's beyond words the scope that these 10 months has for you. Be forgiving and accepting as each change unfolds.

The three c's Calm confident and in control are the under lay of birthing babies. When you are calm confident and in control, it seems like the everything. When you are calm confident and in control, you always have control, not of the environment necessarily but you have control of your mind and your body and how you respond to the environment. Your thoughts and the way the chemical makeup of your body responds to the environment. Not just to birth your baby but to make life forward the way you want it. You have this silent power. It's a palpable strength you have when you remain calm.

You have the choices you have the bond you have the beautiful bond with baby. And it supports you in staying calm confident and in control and making sure your intentions and needs through the progression of your life are fulfilled.

You have the unique bond with your baby that no one will ever know, your partner will have their own connection with you and with baby but the love between you and your body and your ability to birth baby is immeasurable and incomparable.

Your baby is grown within you, you don't need to tell your body how to do it because it already knows.

You maybe require reminder occasionally that you do know what to do, just like your body knows what to do. You will experience the simple fleeting acceptances within you every cell of your body aligning with it's natural purpose and growing baby, without thought purposefully guiding you to nutrients and actions and internal and external actions support mechanisms that will nourish baby within you. It is astounding, we don't even think it down to this level. You have it. You are it. A complete life support unit for a growing human. And it's host. If that doesn't inspire you to believe in yourself I don't know what will.

You are growing the cellular connections that will support your baby for the whole nine months, more so, it's entire life, and prepare your body for birthing baby. In the early pregnancy days it's natural to feel tired it's a tiredness you will have never known but it is called growth. You are establishing the infrastructure to sustain, so much. Knowing you were born with the ability to immaculately build this infrastructure is incredible, in and of itself. Latent until you need it. Much like many inherent assets you have. So were guiding you through the fascinating latencies of your body, into a confident birth.

Having babies and parenting are one of the most challenging and rewarding experiences of your life.

When you lean your attention towards what it is that you would like to happen, using the inclusive scripts and maybe purchasing the audios, reading these pages and allowing yourself to learn new ways, you are more likely to change the way life unfolds to change the way your pregnancy unfolds. Were all aware of what could go right and what could go wrong, here you are Unlocking a path of what could go rightness more easily. You turn more of the what could go rightness into your life. And you can be confident enough to trust that if there is a go wrongness you can turn it into a go rightness very quickly with the flick of a thought and a turn of your intention. And what you learn will begin to become automatic.

Your unlocking opening, a path of what could be and what can happen. In this book there will be facts and ideas and principles you already know. Without turning into a tree hugging earth mother. The science of birth and the innate essence and capability of your body. The natural rhythm and the innate essence in you that enables you to captivate your focus and personal choices and make them so. To work with your body and work with the foundations of who you are. To use hypnotherapy for child birth to birth your baby confidently. There are some, really simple facts that you may or may not know but will make complete sense to you as your read them. You will find a natural alignment within you for everything here, it will just sit right with you if you choose. And form a layer of strength and confidence. To birth your baby with ease and to birth your baby with love. And to enjoy the experience of labour and birth.

This text works alongside the medical professionals who are engaged with you through your pregnancy, journey. The medical aspect including your midwife and Obstetrics practitioners domain.

Your beliefs will change. Your experience will change. Your flexibility will change. Things will change but they will change so subtly that you won't even notice you will just change. Something that will awaken your inner sense inner guide and inner support network which is so much more potent and powerful than you can possibly imagine. You will very quietly awaken. The natural instincts you have will strengthen the natural insight of the woman who often remains silent dormant, the power that is within your will very gently awaken to strengthen you.

It's so much more active than you can imagine and more beautiful than you can believe. But it's only when we look to the possibility, set fears aside and just allow the time to dream and explore the possibility of what can be to the positive. What can become. What you and your body can actually be capable of. What you are actually capable within your thoughts, within your body and how something very simple to change can make a huge rolling impact in your life moving forward. Allot of the principles in this book will spread out in waves through your life like ripples.

Birthing baby can be a very powerfully positive experience. It can feel good. Women aren't sold this image by the media but it's the real truth. Labour does not have to be laboric.

By allowing yourself the space to think about what you want, what can go right and also being prepared for the inevitable things don't always go right. And have a solution there already lined up ready to present itself at the right time. Birthing babies will give you the feeling of control. The point in principle is when you are pregnant it is a place of vulnerability. But also great strength. There are so many unknowns the most common feeling of being led by the system is very very common. The truth is you can follow the system work with the system and also have your own plan. Birthing babies strengthens your plan. Makes your plan more plausible, more possible and more real. It gives you control. You can't always control what happened around you, you can't always control everything and nor should you seek to. But you have the ability to control how you respond to what happens and always turn that in a positive experience.

You are in control of and that's what's important. This is your birth. Your baby your experience. We may not be able to change you the physiology of your body but you will uncover how to work best with what it has. And that is a skill you will have forever.

This path, using the birthing babies book and audios will enable you to build confidence and calm, when you appreciate you are building and maintain an incubation and life support system which is perfectly ordinated. Which means you are control of the vibrational, load that baby receives from you. Functionally physically your body is doing miraculous job of managing the nutrients baby needs from you without even thinking, so if you think that the genetics and the innate lines of physicality and instinct, in the same way as the natural order that breathes baby, nourishes baby and grows you, your womb your muscular structures , has more intelligence to birth baby, than we have been encouraged to believe you would be correct. You are one loop, with a current and flow between you and your unborn baby, are nurturant in more ways than just nutritional, your thoughts emotions and feelings influence baby. The beauty of birthing babies is it enables you to stay calm build confidence release fears and to enjoy the building excitement towards your birth.

The science of birth can be intimidating. We fear the genetics of birth and development in case they presume to us imperfection or deformity. Science does not hinder us, but sometimes when we know more, there is more to process more to fear. Beware the trap that depends too much on science, than listening to your instincts. They can both coexist in balance but the way the balance is perceived in balance sometimes needs to be reset. So we can equally celebrate the origins of childbirth.

Things don't always go well and things don't always go to plan...and that's not always ok but the one thing you can always do is own it unless you own it you cant change it. Your mind your feelings your experiences your fears your thoughts. All of it.

The most important thing is resilience and personal strength. We aren't installing here, you are being reminded you already have it but you might not have seen it in this way before.

Either way it's useful because then you know you have it when you need it. Because you are enough. Even and most especially when it doesn't feel like it.

Draining and refueling - Pregnancy can feel draining. But it doesn't need to be if you imagine draining isn't the concept, it isn't even the word. You are building. It takes a change in perspective growing a baby does not drain you it focusses you on what is important. And that is just different and takes your energy inside.

You are building, that takes energy but you can rest. You are being nourished by baby in prospect, with potential and future hopes as you are nourishing baby with nutrients and life. There are no drains. It's all nourishment. The hopes should as you move forward through birthing babies be lighter, less burdensome instead of have to's they become " can do's " and " love to's ".

You are learning to balance feminine strength with assertion,

Femininity is a strange thing. It's subjective, including a mix of vulnerability, beauty and graceful strength. Having the confidence to assert what you intend for your body and your baby is not always easy. By doing and not doing and striking a balance that protects and preserves you both. The deal is that the true confidence and the essence of you as a woman is inherent. Turning the aspect into the context of galvanising your birth plan - to gently assert your strength without the pressure of conformity, or over assertion is important.

Non exclusively for the fathers out there it's true also evolving and opening up the sense of humility and appreciation for the women there before you. Carrying your own thoughts fears and apprehensions and expectations, your responsibility as a supporter, a rock, a father the best version of a father you can imagine, becoming that take acknowledgement too. Together becoming incredible parents. Both, together and as individuals. If you are a lone parent doing pregnancy alone, then even more so you centre your support and become stronger. Strong enough for two.

Just like you are the support system for baby, you now mirror that in life. Support is crucial sometimes and when it does not appear to your from external sources it's because you have it inside. With each and every step of pregnancy and birth and beyond you want to feel supported, at some level some how and some way you want to feel competent you want to feel confident and if you don't want to now there are times in the future you will definitely want to feel these things. The thing is that these things come from inside of you and recognition is required. We often seek these outside of ourselves but, you accept that on some level the most important asset you have is you. Your need to seek, comfort, approval, diminishes and are within you that recognition is required.

As you move through these pages thoughts and ideas will unlock and enable you to build stronger new alliances. Because when you think about it there is only one person you can really rely on for support ever ... and that's you.

you can feel confident

you can feel supported

You can feel heard

You can feel loved.

Consistently

You can support you by allowing yourself to over come fears and become. Quite often pregnancy brings baby brain, brings clumsiness brings all of the things that undermine you, brings our weaknesses up as well as our strengths. Because you are growing a human. When the majority of your energy is directed inside to the growing baby and infrastructure of support building within you. It takes effort to be. To show interest to be interested and it's natural to feel the strain. But also to be aware means it is no longer a strain but an acceptance. So you can be present and aware.

Letting yourself evolve as the best version of a mother or father that you can be. It isn't about thinking yourself into capability, it's reminding yourself into capability, being capable. You can think it, you can shout it from the rooftops what you are, used to be, and how others were with you, but your real intention is in your thoughts and actions. The thoughts and actions of you. Because that determines you. We look at the word determine as a forward force determined action, but you can intend and then determine, that is how life becomes by moving with your intentions. It can be gentle and graceful.

Wherever there is incapability there is hidden capability behind it. Accept the wobbles and believe they are strengthening you. Just as so. Wherever there is insufficiency there is sufficiency behind it. So wherever you are weaknesses, there are strengths incumbent, not brave enough there is strength within and behind it. Wherever you have not enough ness there is a hidden enoughness within you. That has been lain dormant. Not loved enough, not confident enough.. There is always a comparison which means you have the very thing you wanted within you but you just haven't uncovered it yet to it's full potential. Sometimes it feels like the world is moving you, but that changes when you learn and start moving it aswell. You see it differently. Just like wearing sunglasses, your filters change.

Example, Today I'm wearing my confident lenses, (filters) and you embody the confidence. Like a favourite outfit, your lucky pants, but something you wear on the inside, because it becomes you. So bright that it has a visible discernable hue.

It's just about the turn of perspective, with anything it's just about the turn of perspective. Where you feel unloved, you have the hidden capacity to be loved in the perfect way for you. You just have not activated it yet. You must have it within you otherwise you would not know how to not have it.

Wherever you feel lacking there is something you aren't yet and that is what is missing, it's just a matter of time and it will all fall into place. It's here waiting ready to become you. Maybe you haven't even discovered it yet the space for it but when the space is there you will naturally fill it and unfold into it it to become the person you had the space to become. That's how it happens. You unfold and you grow as a person. You know this already.

That means overcoming your own hang ups and your fears about child birth. When you let the fear be known then it can be healed. Overcome and released. When youre searching for something it will elude you then when you let it go, it makes space for it to appear. Then it can.

When youre on your everyday path it will be there, ready ahead of you to become you.

For you, for your partner, and most of all for baby and your future together. As a partner or a lone parent or for a life with a future partner. That sounds like a pretty big ask for a book about hypnotherapy and childbirth but it is so much more than that. It's a style of living that, and fundamental evolution in the way you think, in which you are able to choose what your life will entail.

If you can grow and nurture an entire human being naturally then you can make sure you are fully engaged with the joy.

It's a fundamental shift in your beliefs about what your body is capable of and how your beliefs and thoughts about child birth can shift very deeply very quickly just by education.

It's opening your eyes to different perspectives that will challenge and change you and enable you to grow easily with each and every shift.

And that's why.

You can form new and exciting constellations of happiness, of belief and possibility, new networks of support and new networks of inspiration. New networks whatever networks you are missing out on. But you don't know they're missing until you think about it. Until you reflect. Until you try something new and then you realise that you did not know how good it would be until you tried it and then you want more. That's expansion. And that's ok.

Whatever those constellations are, support, friendship, business, all of the ways you life will grow through motherhood. Let it grow and you grow with it. Having the confidence to grow and the ability to hold those aspects of pregnancy, birth and mother hood (parent hood) is going to unfold.

In thinking these they will become something and the more you intend them consciously, enjoy them and embrace them the more they become a something. Your thoughts are intentions and will turn into somethings whether they are what you want or not, so learning to tame the fears and fine tune your intentions by intending what you really do love and really do want to happen is a necessary undercurrent moving forward. Once again we don't know what were doing until we check it. So check it, if it's good do it, if it isn't change it.

It sounds like large expectations, but looking forward ten years and thinking backwards you will be grateful that you read this book. You will notice (and probably forget this sentence until some time in the future when your reminded and then you will notice how many different shifts and changes have happened how your perspectives changed) You might even find the book and think what did this even do for me because it became you already. It's that powerful.

And if at this point you are thinking, I don't know if I can go on because this is really airy fairy book, hard to get into, It's designed that way so keep going. The lead page says chapter 1. (The boring bit) Intros, ground work, like the house keeping section of a training. Keep reading.

Using hypnosis for child birth is easy.... It's simple. It works under the surface. I'm not saying that you can birth a baby without any effort at all. But the effort to use Hypnotherapy for child birth is outweighed immensely by promise it holds for therapeutic change.

The effort isn't effort, it isn't mental effort, you don't push a baby out of your vagina with your head.

You control your thoughts and redirect them in a way that moves your energy to calming your body and your body then progresses the birth of baby with you calm confident and in control. You birth a baby with your mental control of your attention, so that your attention brings calm to your body and your mind and the body can then birth baby as it was naturally designed to do. You do that unconsciously. You birth baby by being present, by consciously breathing, and being present in the moment which Hypnotherapy for childbirth and birthing babies enables you to do. If you are not present you are afeared, when you are calm you are present because the fears are allayed. So birthing babies, It just makes you more efficient. Efficiency is everything.

You are birthing baby, using hypnosis for childbirth means you can be present because the ground work is preloaded within your mind. You don't need to think about it and that's why it's so beautiful.

That is not to say child birth is easy.

My learning over time is that as adults thinking minds we think too much. Thinking has it's place, but when we think about things it overcomplicates them. Thinking in the right way is important. It's all about efficiency so are your thoughts refining, feel your thoughts refining. If you think about alchemy, in the refinement of your thoughts and the expenditure of your attention. The quality of your attention and intention changes. Becomes clearer, more beautiful. Efficiency is relative to time. Time is one of the most precious commodities we have, and we spend it where it is most effective, with efficacy, and with alignment with our hearts. It has a different quality. When we think and become distracted, it becomes dilute. Fractionated. Allow the worries to subside. Allow what is not important to just be. And instead appreciate this moment of everything being ok.

Like you didn't think about that until you thought about it and once you thought about it, it became important - that's only for the good things. Obsess about the things you love. The things you enjoy the things you aspire to privately or openly.

The thoughts about the things that are uncertain the uncontrollables, the things that stop us in our tracks unnecessarily. That is something you will find through the whole of this book. When thinking stops. You start living. There is a place for thinking planning and there is a place for experiencing Physically, energetically, You have what I call the centre a center line. Where your personal strength and congruence it is. The stronger you get with determination, the more obvious this is. We have a heart mind alignment, and when you sway, to assess the other options, when your thinking from side to side in your eyes, in your mind weighing up the options of the people and the time and the....Whatever ... it takes you off your centerline. It's like the place where you gut instinct is. All the silent ripples in the atmosphere and environment that your inner mind is aware of but doesn't necessarily alert you to. They may rise as a side eye fear misrepresented in a different context though it is likely something overcommable when you trust.

Imagine your centre line is where you know. And it's ok to express it and it is ok to know it even silently. It's often silent but when you knowing of your centre line. Were building a stronger centre line here now. Imagine your yes nose and heart stomach. That the place of alignment and congruence. Have you ever heard the term easily swayed. That is the heart mind alignment in challenge. Your working on your core... and I promise no sit ups required yet.

When you are centred it's all right there (well center) it is all there inside aligned and perfected. It's all there with an inner strength that grows and grows ... the more you use it the more it grows. The more you fill it. The more you learn. The more you know about you, the world, what you want is to embellish it.

So whatever you do not know consciously there will be a hue moving through you making the fears and worries dissolve the more you align with your center line. Your instinct the place you are aware of the all, the millions and millions of filtered perceptions of the reality you are living in calculated on the strength of everything you are not aware of which if you knew about it thought about it consciously would absolutely blow you away. These perceptual filters change when you evolve, learn, let things go and realign your motivation and desires. Making you more determined, more consistent and more invested.

There will always be a sway. But it will sway you less. It's like to core of you sits centre, and when we don't know what to do we sit either side, but when you are discerned and committed you are centre and strong. In times of challenge or trauma it is different. (wait until chapter 7)

Some of the things we want to avoid will send us off that line, fears, worries past experiences may send us into a different saturation. But you learn to strengthen your central set point so you have a central always know what to do, residing in you.

Thinking is helpful and has it's place but when thinking is a worry-based fear based pattern. Knowing is different and developing the self trust to know is something that comes with practice. It comes as you read. You have it already, if you have it already fantastic. For others it comes with time and practice. But like a rainbow sometimes when you keep looking for it, it will elude you. It's something you are, not something you can find and seek.

We spend too much time complicating things so much so sometimes that the solutions don't come. So much so that we block the solutions by over thinking. It becomes clear later in the book.

So hypnotherapy and guided relaxation helps, it opens up the very place in you where the out of this world solutions are found, where you have more control than you ever imagined. Because very simply, you expand your consciousness in alignment with the suggestion of the guide, then you return. Each time you expand it deepens the change a little more. This is called fractionation.

Hypnosis is about guided relaxation and visualisation our intention is more easily accessible to our minds when we engage with relaxation and the creative spirit. Building a familiarity and rapport with the you in you. You begin to make things happen that are for you.

Indulge your imagination, the possible and the impossibles may become less impossible.

The relaxations states enable you to gently access your inner mind your unconscious mind and it's potency in rapport. As you use them more you became attuned to your unconscious mind and it will work with you more as you become aware and relax and follow that inner instinct. But making it very simple.

Where you can potentialize anything and allow it to unfold, so potentializing what it is that you love and what you would like to go right is the key when you really embody the love you feel for having children - you can handle it all.

"Having Kids feels like that first seventh-grade crush that overwhelms every molecule in your body, but it's permanent. – Kristen Bell "

It will be less burdensome the constant feeling of it. You can just embody the love for them.

So as you listen to the audios and work your way through the book they will merge with your Knowledge and become you. In a very subtle way. It will change the perceptions of who you are an what you do, very subtly.

The relaxations states enable you to gently access your inner mind your unconscious mind and it's potency in rapport. As you use them more you became attuned to your unconscious mind and it will work with you more as you become aware and relax and follow that inner instinct. But making it very simple.

It feels good.

It's good for your body to rest restore and reset in relaxation sessions The series of Audio downloads available for a nominal investment. Via The ' online training' Tab at www.victoriawhitney.com. 6 twenty or so minute relaxation sessions which perfectly complement birthing babies. The are powerful. But there are only 1000 copies available per year so get yours now. Several relaxation sessions are noted in this book. record them and listen.

It's interesting, learning about your body and a your mind, almost expansion of what you are capable of just by intending it.

Builds your confidence. Makes things effortless - Not by expectation but be reflection. Have benefits we don't even know about yet ... filters out through your whole life.

It actually filters out through your life, underlays confidence and a sense of composure across your life. Makes you stronger and more easily able to recognize and assert your wishes, dreams and desires.

It underlays new and more fulfilling perception eliminates self-doubt and increases your confidence in being you.

Builds your bond with baby – strengthens the connection you have with baby and strengthens the connections you have with your natural wishes and desires for you, pregnancy, birthing and beyond. And all of the other things.

When you think about it this is life now.... Moving forward will be a whole new way of being a whole new life for you. A birth of another human being and a full time evolution of your family. If you are a lone parent doing pregnancy alone and building a future for you and baby that is brave, and it will build your strength in assertion to unfold the best life you can muster for baby and in the moments you feel less than enough there will be a resounding internal cheerleader strengthening you for within whether or not you have the support from loved ones from the people around you or whether you are committed to taking pregnancy through alone. And even opening up the space for your match to enter your life.

It gives you that priceless you time, when you and baby are working towards labour together when you are listening to the audios.

When you are at the end of the day ... like you have given enough the day is done and you are craving something and you don't know what it is this is the time to turn to the audios, and taking some time to rest restore and relax. Those 30 minutes of listening tuning into you and baby will be reward some through the whole of your life. The intention is that everything in the book can be applied in many ways.

Your mind is also incredibly powerful and can form new and positive connections with great ease. Just by intending it so and giving yourself permission. It means you can under the surface create new resources, new opportunities just by reading you will make new connections and associations and your perspectives on life and what Is possible for you, birth baby and beyond being possible. It allows the fears to lift. It allows for a sense of calm inside and allows for the internal security to flow forward and to feel a sense of joy and excitement a sense of calm and happiness.

You will be inspired and enlightened by the simplest of things and they will like constellations form new connections moving forward. Everywhere you go there will be new meetings, support, coincidences just because you changes the way you thought, you changed your trajectory. The trajectory of your mind. Learning anything does this. The trajectory of your acceptance and of so many things.

It's about acceptance, acceptance of yourself, acceptance of what is and acceptance of your ability to change and influence the way things are.

You say determined, but right now, strength is in intending, and intending to determine with your mind. Determination precedes and speaks to action, but also to inaction. Determined to or not to, because you are doing something this way. You are confident, you are in control and you intend to birth your baby with confidence. Fully committing, intending, determining the intention you have beyond that birth.

It's different, see it. Your intentions are quite often silent, they are strength they are you. You intend with each thought each word and each breath and you intend well.

Each of these being an old action, idea or limitation turning into a new possibility with solutions which don't need to be finite. When what is at the core is your mission your vision and intention and support to that intention.

You are becoming more of you; you will recognize strengths you didn't even know you had. You will open new portals of insight and imagination and also unfold in ways you haven't imagined. Your perceptions and experience of pregnancy and childbirth will change as you allow yourself and your pregnancy to unfold. With possibility. That you can birth with ease and minimise discomfort but more than that that you can make a greater life beyond birth too.

In some ways you are willing to change your perceptions and open your mind to new possibilities and thought streams that will be different and new to you. That's ok, you can accept what is right for you and then the rest let it wash over you like water of a ducks back.

Inoculating yourself from the words of others when they don't serve you when they don't really feel like they are yours or would work for you. They will just wash over you like water of a ducks back.

What is reasonable and what is appropriate where there are risks it is important that they are addressed in a way that is appropriate that the professionals that are around you will be supportive and identify risk where they present and take appropriate action Pregnancy should be something that is a beautiful experiences a joy and a new beginning. And the tiny excitements about each. From the very First scans .Everything is so much more real. Seeing that image on screen for the first time is something so beautiful. So much more real. You can fully be enveloped in the miracles that you are growing within your womb. Sometimes it is intimidating for some to invest such hope when they have experienced Trauma or loss. You see it and it is really there. It becomes so much more real. The baby becomes a more real because it is not just a concept or a hope or a line on a test when you can see their picture. It becomes more real. You feel the connection.

It's really there it's moving and breathing and it's tiny heart beating. Everything becomes much more, baby moves, you see baby moving for the first time!

These are the once in a lifetime moments. To enjoy. Allowing your faith to build and fears to subside you can fully enjoy each and every moment.

Even when you have multiple babies each one has it's own personality, and temperament which is discernible even from the womb. The profile of their face you will find will carry through their lives with them. When you see the sideways profile photo. And then remember to look back in 5 or 10 years time their profile will not have changed in it is size yes but design no. It is extraordinary. When you are experiencing the pregnancy symptoms. You can choose to embrace the love or you can choose to embrace the discomfort. Choose to JFDI or choose to grumble. You can grumble but really when you check yourself and think about it even when you have the heart burn and the kicks and finding it difficult to position in sleep, and you haven't started maternity leave yet and you have to be at work in the morning and can't sleep, you can't really grumble. You can laugh about it, because you remember. It's only a matter of time. Before you meet your baby, and every discomfort you experienced in pregnancy will fade into insignificance. From around 20 week there is evidence that baby can hear your voices. So you can even use your voice to bond with baby. Baby can hear what you hear. You would be careful what you said if someone was listening from outside the door. So every sentiment you give your baby, is based on something good. Getting the best start, just like you take your pre natal vitamins. Take your daily relaxation session. And experience that sense of calm that you are being looked after by something kind, because it's you.

Imagine it from babies perspective. What a way to start out in life. How to install a faith in a world worth living in. Maybe baby will birth easier just by having the sense that the journey down the birth canal is taking them to a new kind of eutopia. If a place sounds good you would be more willing to make the journey. And make it quick and easy!

They really want to get here because it sounds so good. Every day is a blessing. It's not without challenge you will have days. Up days down days, that is life. It's how you deal with those days that's most promising. Here you are galvanising your core. In all of the ways. You were a you ... and now an us. Baby and you. In that simple moment so much can change. And it is all good (even if it isn't) Believe it enough and it will. (as long as you don't start rainbow chasing and looking for the magic.) The magic is you. That is the whole point.

Physically the mechanics – youre going to grow and you are going to grow some more. The average woman gains around 22 to 28 pounds body weight. Your body and your make up will change in way that are known but unknown and ways that are seen and unseen and ways that may shake you and ways that will make you. You will still love your body. Be more forgiving of it. Because it is doing something amazing.

When it can't move so fast and when you feel so huge that you waddle. It is only a matter of time.

There is nothing so beautiful than the feeling of baby moving and the sight of your pregnant belly becoming bigger and bigger filled with life. Moving around and feet sticking out this way when they kick. To proceed with confidence. You are going to be silently empowered, because when you are silently empowered you aren't wearing it on your sleeve like a jacket or a badge saying I AM EMPOWERED, because it begs them to ask ..." come show me then." It's like a battle call sometimes. That's not always a helpful invitation. Pick your battles and save your energy. Most times staying in your power resisting the temptation to overstep, brag and instigate what may be a battle, that you have already won because you are it, is the better way. Simply embody the love. The empowerment.

Building determination and the assertion to communicate your choices. Easier said than done to some. The thing is when you are confident in your choices as you are becoming, it's easier to communicate them. When your heart strength is invested in you it's easier to make those choices and communicate those choices in a calm and diplomatic way. And when required within your power you are more than welcome to get your bitch on. You are supported. You know your body and you know when something is right or wrong and you just know. You're getting to know your body more and more and it is fascinating. It's capable of creating life. That's not a nothing, that's a something.

We are taught how to fear birth taught to fear the strength of a woman and her assertion of will, taught to rely and not be independent in choice and determination of intention. We are taught how to birth we are taught to lie down and push. To be static. All these layers of learning are just there waiting to be changed, educated into something different. Because that is not the only way. Before we progress.. an important and responsible point.

The general trend in Hypnotherapy for child birth is often the intent on birthing baby naturally with minimal intervention. In recent times in 2022 there has been investigations into hospital ignorance about the amount of people recommending natural birth when intervention would have saved lives, lives of mothers and lives of babies. Countless lives have been saved by the use of hypnosis in child birth because labours progress more easily. There is always a counter point though and the only solution to inoculate yourself from a potential mistake is to be attentive to you and your body and to weigh the advice of professionals on Your inteligence and balance what is instinctively right for you. If you need help. Get help.

The thing is, noone would want for a clinical intervention such as forceps, episiotomy or venteuse, if they did not need it. No one wants that. The interference unless it is necessary and lifesaving. What you want is to birth your baby. As you choose, from a faith standpoint rather than a fear. If clinical intervention is required you still birthed your baby and can be confident that you did do everything in your ability to contribute to the birth you wanted. Even if it did not work out that way. You can still use the principles to remain calm confident and in control no matter what.

To be strong enough to accept that intervention may be required and accept that that is ok. And to be calm confident and in control no matter what. Acceptance that it is all part of the journey because the real reason will come after. The silver lining, the bright side. If something happens it usually happens for a reason. Accepting intervention or that you may not have the birth experience you had planned takes great strength. But in acceptance is the ability to change your perspective, and accept that the priority may shift to preserving the lives of you and baby and whatever that takes is ok. There is only pride in that. What is most important is the health and lives of you and baby and with that in mind it isn't defeat.

So many women report a sense of failure when natural births don't take place as planned that tends to linger in people ... It is never a failure. As a hypnotherapist it is easy for me to say that this course, this book, this text and the audios, will give you everything you need inside to birth your baby with confidence that does not mean you must birth your baby without any form of intervention or any form of medication. It means you will birth your baby with confidence whether this requires intervention or not. And acceptance of how it happens because the one thing you will be is calm, confident and in control, And feel proud to yourself for having done so.

As you are enough, to accept intervention in success, if it saves your life or the life of baby. Being enough sometimes means being enough to ask for help and to accept it.

And to keep the feeling of accomplishment, as if you had breathed every single contraction everything you had practiced, and it all went perfectly. Because what you did do was, in most cases more brave.

One thing women do not find easy is assertion. What is assertion anyway. Quite often women remain unheard unable to express what they want. It's quite streight forward. Very gently it is possible to assert oneself, ones intention with a grace that is somehow very assuring. Assertion by shouting dominating, not required, when you start with a gentle determined, then if it gets you no where you can build up to the other means. Assertion means making sure you are at the top of the list and that you ask the questions, you want to ask with confidence, the uncomfortable questions. You ask the uncomfortable questions. You're not a nothing or a noone in the face of an expert you are a someone and a very important something.

So you underlay it. The self worth. Your self worth. every day you build a little bit more by respecting yourself and complimenting you.

The real origins of motherhood are very far removed from how you birth your baby directly they are an instinct, through labor and childbirth and were here at the dawn of man, we have evolved over centuries. They began to confuse the evolution of medical science with an override of nature. That science is great and knows best. The medicine medicalisation is a crucial factor, But it's Not THE crucial factor. It's an enhancement not a replacement. To revisit origins.

The last two hundred years a Transition from natural birthing into assisted birthing. Where this has become the norm. Our aim. To consider birth without fear. To consider the revision of that back step and take a step forwards.

Medicalisation, is good when something goes wrong, but also exists the path of what could go right and the possibilities for reduced medicalisation. We are taught how painful birth is, we see in the movies women screaming and the episodes on one born every minute (which I love) are always presenting the same image that women – and birth it is loud. It's painful. Drugs help and that it is dramatic. All these layers to learn new through.

The thing I learned and that you are learning now is that they only televise the births that are dramatic and that are dramatic and the ones that are uncomfortable and will make the best TV the most riveting watching and entertainment purposes.

The ones that will keep people coming back to the TV shows that will have people immersed in watching through to the end of the programme, will be shown.

If someone walked in, Silent, with twinkly music, relaxed calm, elegant, silent and within 2 -3 hours breezed in breathed, smiled and then squeezed a baby out, poker faced in a birthing pool with bliss music and a smile on her face. Then held baby for the photo, (insta - obviously) got out had a shower dressed in their pre pregnancy jeans, and went home with a sleeping content baby. They would not show it because it's not entertainment. It is fascinating, jaw dropping. But it wouldn't make TV. It is amazing to experience. That is possible. That is power. That could be you. If it is what you want. If you want drama. Put the book down and walk away.

It is all about the perspective appreciating what is possible. We have a preconceived perception of what pushing is like, what we are sold is a sedentary birth.

I remind you. Your experience is unique every one experience is unique.You can choose how you experience it. You may not be able to choose how events transpire but you can choose the way you experience them.

Moving baby through the birth canal is your bodys role. You are just showing up for the day to oversee the process.

Your breath and support your body by nourishing it with helpful feelings and thoughts, by staying calm it has the opportunity to continue to flow the hormones that progress labour and actively inhibit pain.

It takes the endurance out of the process because it becomes a journey of a moment at a time one contraction at a time one breath at a time which eventually will lead you to a final push and the birth of baby. Just one step at a time.

Day by day building the structures the cellular structures in your body that will assist you in birthing baby that strengthen the physical muscular pathways and also the mental pathways they will all work together. Your learning you will be making new associations and new future memories and new future choices, every day of your pregnancy something grows a little bit more, in your body, and that can be mirrored in your life, something becomes a firmer plan, more certain, more solid. It's all there solidifying before you and you are now a participant in your life moving forward. A participant with choice. And the power to make it the way you want it. You have choice you have strength and you are going to use it. Read on. Learn some more about how amazing you actually are.

And build the confidence to birth your baby with ease.

We are helping you to establish firm confidence in you and who you are to establish the sentiment of who you are and you full alignment with creating the life you want for you and your family.

It will be there inside when you need it most.

You are just here to be reminded of everything you already are, but didnt know yet. Thats what you need inside to birth your baby with confidence and ease and overcome any challenge in life moving forward.

(not a big ask)

BIRTHING BABIES - TOP TIPS

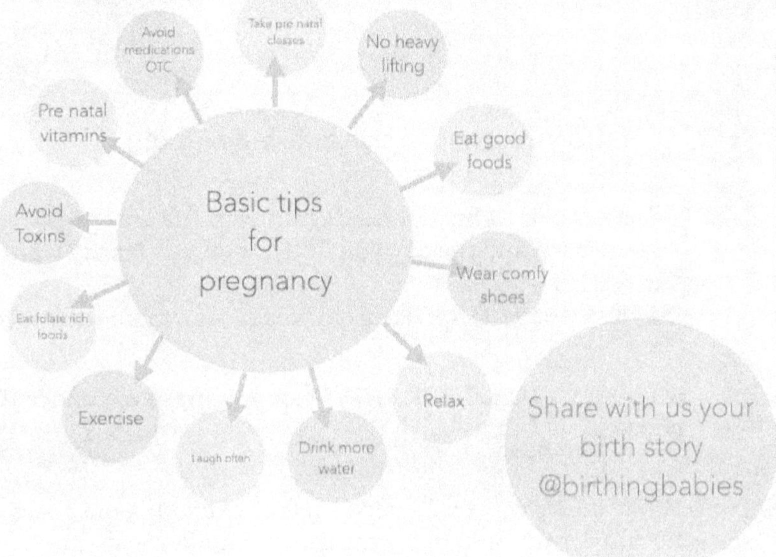

CHAPTER 2

" Do you want to dance like a chicken ... "

"The two most important days in your life are the day you
are born and the day you find out why." – Mark Twain

Do you want to dance like a chicken ... As a hypnotherapist.

SO MANY PEOPLE ASK THIS " can you make me dance like a
chicken"

What do I say... Yes... but I charge extra. It's old news and
no fun for me. Making great things happen is so much more
fulfilling.

In context. People often ask me can you make me dance
like a chicken. Yes I can, If you would dance like that after
a bottle of wine or few vodkas then yes. BUT. See this a
different way. In context of childbirth. The chicken dance,
comes from TV, What else has come from TV, what you
have been brainwashed to believe is a reality in life, AKA (in
context) painful birth is completely unnecessary and a very
different kind of hypnosis. With a very different intention
within it. All tender hot chicken dancing is ineffectual use of
the real value of a very powerful process. To work for greater
good. Chicken dancing. It is funny but not really after the first
time..... So rather than being entranced by the media. The TV
and all the stories of how hard birth is you can choose your
own and believe in a more helpful suggestive installation.

Your now. You are going to be birthing a baby.

You have a plan for that birth.

You want to be educated (or you're bored so your reading, and
pregnant so you feel it should be something baby related).

You want to influence the birth of your child.

Directly - Hypnotherapy, for child birth. It sounds like a process but it is more an experience. To the hypnotherapist it is a process to you the subject, or active participant you are the owner of your experience of the process. Including enjoying your body, enjoying being pregnant and enjoying being alive. In order to experience it and really experience it you don't need to think about it. It something you experience it is your experience and it feels good.

Why would you even go there. You have your own reasons which you can list .... Do it now.

There are so many reasons that I can give you. But they are mine, yours will be different. I love it. So it is a no brainer, and I have seen it work, thousands of times.

But this is for you. I can tell you why, but you have your own reasons and they are the most compelling. You want your reasons because that is your why. That is s your mojo. Your forward motion. Your purpose. That is your why.

To get you started I share.. To use it, to do and to have it, to see other people after they have been through it and come through the other side. All of the joys. Thats my why. Whats yours.

(When I used it for child birth, to have a low chemical birth was my aim. That was my why. Yours will inevitably be different.)

Here are some reasons from a professional opinion to get you started. Why would you want to use Hypnotherapy for child birth...

It feels good
It is comfortable
It is relaxing
Its enjoyable.
It moves your mind in places to make good things happen. It

builds a sense of connection with you and your inner mind. It makes the most difficult things and concepts seem simple straight forward and easy

It makes it possible to do things that seemed previously difficult or snaggy. It encourages your body to be more relaxed, and greater health comes from that sense of greater relaxation. Replenishes your body and your nervous system by centering you inside so the distractions become less as you attune more to your real self within. Restores your connection with yourself. Increases your internal uptake of serotonin and dopamine encouraging a generally feeling of wellbeing and happiness. You can increase your pain tolerance – reduce your experience of pain and turn it into discomfort and movement Reduces the activity of the dorsal anterior cingulate cortex. Which is responsible for alertness and vigilance.

This should give you an on off switch to stimulation. You eventually get to choose when you become excited and when you don't but excitement is not of nervousness they are different it becomes a confident excitement.

When you think about your vigilance being responsive to exterior demands and stimulus or as an internal drive to get something, that is causing hypervigilance to an extreme hypnosis will bring that to centre. So it is more harmonised, Your needs, your alertness your internal navigation, based on all of the filters and perceptions of all of the everything you are aware off. It's a sense that is alight for go getting, is it something you desire compared to something you fear. Hypnosis induces you to give you innermind more airtime. So your neurological experience will become more balanced. And your body is more attuned to the inner rhythm and the outer calls are less so. But still present to you can balance your senses to your outer environment in a way that supports you.

Hypnosis will refine your focus and make things more easy. This is how to strengthen the core, beliefs core, "I am" beliefs. Your core without the sit ups.

This enables you to centre, and then anything that wasn't requiring the vigilance it did before becomes less important for your nervous system to seek and track. That's what people find exhausting. This way you are diverted to what is now important which will be different. And then will build a new track. As this track becomes more used it becomes more refined and more functional so these new thoughts and lines of attention that your body and mind will build through the book and through using hypnosis in the written inductions and spoken inductions downloadable will strengthen and becomes permanent filters that are effective through all facets of life in a helpful way.

So you are enabled to refocus your day, your moment your mind and the direction of your energy and the trajectory of your life.

Dependent on the suggestions and purpose for the hypnotherapy.

It's directed guidance and diversion of your attention so as to make good something in your life that was previously not good, so that your attention can bring about more of your desired experiences. It reduces the stress on your body from the repetitive thoughts and sensations that which you can control more easily with a centred mind. Bringing centredness. Working on the core.

This some have shown can reduce the likelihood of unnecessary intervention and increase the efficacy and efficiency of intervention when it is required.

If your birth plan requires intervention like a planed c section it can increase the speed within which you heal and increase the efficacy of the intervention required it can also brings acceptance and joy to the place where you had previously had a heart set on a natural birth.

That's what I mean by efficacy and efficiency you can intend for the best care and the best choices and the best for you and the best feeling. Assertion balanced with acceptance of what might happen being ok because you are at the centre of it and can confidently move through it with grace, ease and faith.

Does hypnosis change you. Yes but not always as obvious as a chicken dance. Quite often people will recognise something different - you look well today or compliment them on something. Because they can't quite make out what it is but they know something is different.

Sometimes it's almost like you can identify a certain haze about the people I have seen. Like a glow, a hue. It's like a hue of life. Let us call it the Hue. The Hue of confidence, a hue of health, of vibrancy a hue, even if they drink like a fish, eat junk food and smoke 20 a day they will still have this hue. It is like an intactness. Because they do it with love. They are congruent in what they are doing.

A certain intactness that doesn't come around very often, unless your tuned into you. That a result of using hypnotherapy, for personal relaxation. This hue of acceptance of those things we cannot control being slightly more within our control.

It is a faith and trust that comes with strengthening the bond. The place where the hidden layers of worriment and fear can resolve into .... faith. So they are layers of you less conflicted and more at one. That's the sense of the hue. Hypnotherapy brings that hue.

It's all about the Hue. The intactness.

When I meet clients they tend to leave with clear eyes and a hue. That Hue builds between sessions. It grows. I would say an aura but that's different. Because this is a hue. You can do that too with the audios.

With it more specifically with the directed focus on birthing babies, you can increase your pain tolerance – reduce your experience of ' pain " and turn it into discomfort and movement." Increase you confidence as a parent as a woman who can birth. You can turn it into anything.

It's all about the hue - call it lost faith. FOUND.

Recovering togetherness. It's the hue. Get the hue.

If your birth plan requires intervention like a planned c - section it can increase the speed within which you heal and increase the efficacy of the intervention required and make sure you take your hue in there with you. You can have the Hue. It is pre recorded and written in this book so you can speak the relaxation session to yourself.

It can also bring acceptance and joy to the place where you had previously had a heart set on a natural birth. so be it. You can. That's what I mean by efficacy and efficiency you can intend for the best care, the very best choices based on the moment, the very best.

And intend for that to happen and the more you build acceptance with your mind, it will honour your wishes and make paths for these to happen forward, if you just allow yourself to relax and have faith in the process.

It can expand into your life in ways unknown and ways unseen until you are in them and you have a strong faith and confidence.

It's the hue.

You will find it and see it within yourself when you listen to the audios, or record the scripts here in your own voice and listen. A growing hue. That's Assertion of what you would like by intending.

Determining that means just intending it, envisioning it and then relaxing and doing exactly what the relaxation sessions inlay. Balanced with acceptance. That's potent. You can imagine. One that you will be guided by and with on an instinctive level.

Hypnosis has and guided relaxation with suggestive capacity for the non believers been around for centuries.

It Helps you stay focused without being focussed. The hue.

The history of hypnosis is fascinating. And Im a bit of a geek on this kind of thing so humour me.

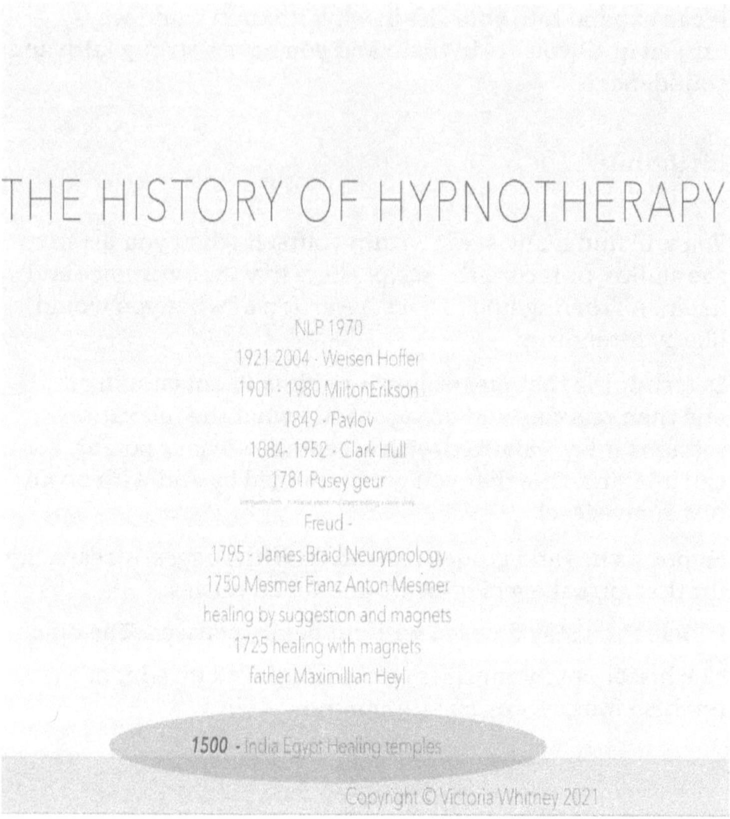

THE HISTORY OF HYPNOTHERAPY

Hypnosis been around forever, beginings in the healing temples in india. It's written in scriptures dating back centuries.

The word Hypnos is the personification of sleep in Greek and again is akin to Sommn in Roman. Also Sommohana part of the yoga vidya - the word somnambulism which is infact sleep walking. From the very begining of time... 350 bc to be precise Aristotle used deep states of relaxation on the encounter of a problem, in one instance, directly with a woman giving birth. I believe the is to be true, even if it isn't on wikipedia. There would be healing caverns, Caverns there would allow people to sleep deep temples like in the pyramids in Egypt it is believed to be very much about tombs and death, but it wasn't just about death, with tombs it was also about the passage of life into death and the healing of life into life the passage and the passage from disease into health.

Europe people believed that Royal touch was healing and example of the power of faith. They didnt know if this was true, but, they believed it true and so it worked. In modern day that's the doctor patient dichotomy that the expert is always the one who has the supreme authority, in past ages just the presence of the professional carries an unconscious expectation to surrender to the power. Though now we are educated and can ask questions we are educated and empowered to answer so the faith in the expert though very present and potent is balanced with the faith of the self in the knowledge you have.

They believed that the hand of the king or queen passes healing through touch. The emphasis of suggestibility in bring about physiological changes. In the bio Rhythm of the body.

In Eurpoe the most memorable and prominent phase of the evolution of hypnotism was mesmer Franz anton mesmer. We have all heard about the mesmeric tendencies mesmeric influences which are universally identified as entrancing.

If you have children already, you probably watch childrens TV in the Uk, Cbeebies and in the night garden is one of the most trance inducing TV programmes I have ever seen. Even now, In a room full of adult health professionals a you tube video that was repetitive, and had no real purpose so the watcher would stay captivated and entranced they couldn't focus on anything else.

Watching someone unpack toys, or watching someone empty cartons of makeup and sprinkle glitter into a pyrex tray through a you tube video was hypnotic and mesmeric. Because your mind is always scanning for purpose. There is no purpose to be found directly only the purpose you find within, which is why it is mesmeric.

It makes no sense, the mind is scanning for way to make it make sense but it doesn't. Its function is to capture attention. And then the mind is open to suggestion, its mesmeric stemming from the legend of Franz Anton Mesmser.

Franz anton Mesmer a german physician with an interest in astronomy. [1]He theorized the existence of an energetic force that crossed between human and inanimate objects and called it animal magnetism.

Later described as mesmerism the polarities of the attractive forces of persuasion. The power of influence.

He used magnets to induce a space of hyper attention and trust and with the attention came a fixation which opened the mind if the person or subject to the suggestion given. So when he passed a magnet over a wound it would heal the would, stop the bleeding, or pass the magnet or object over someones eyes have someone sleep.

Very closely followed by James Braid and Neurypnology - and later termed the phrase hypnotism which is synonymous now with mesmerism . He named this hypnosis after Hypnos, the Greek god of sleep and master of dreams. Around 1847 he identified the phenomena such as anaesthesia and amnesia.

James Esdaile carried forward Mesmerism. He has suffered asthma and bronchitis in his early adolescence and has actively pursued cures. He travelled extensively and settled as civil surgeon at an Indian hospital.

By 1848, a mesmeric hospital supported entirely by public subscription was opened in Calcutta especially for Esdaile's work. It was closed 18 months later by the Deputy Governor of Bengal, Sir John Little. Esdaile was later transferred to the marine surgeon in 1849. If there was no warrant for acknowledgment of benefit ,why would a colonial hospital be established in respect of pain free measures being effective. It must work.

The time line continues on with Leibalt the anaesthesia of suggestion, as an evolution of hypnosis and entered the Nancy school The Nancy school was a hypnotherapy and physiotherapy 1866 supported by Baronheim – The continued mesmerism and animal magnetism, and of course the Label Hypnosis.

Bringing suggestibility to the medical field – this was the real birth of medicine and hypnosis combined but mainly in Europe. The school was successful.

How does this combine with Pshychology and the famous Pshycholgists of all time.

Sigmund Freud.

Freud studied with charcot and resisted Nancy school and the college of hypnosis he was at the time a cocaine addict and had been given wooden teeth this mean his ability to oral dexterity required for hypnotism was limited so he induced and proactively motioned talking cures and catharsis where he would speak very little.

He had palatial cancer and which reduced his ability to articulate. Having undergone many surgeries for cancer yet he still refused to give up smoking.

The evolution alongside hypnosis of Talking therapy with a prediction that it would take – 1-00 to 300 hours to affect a cure.

In modern days significant change can be achieved in lite long conditions of neurosis in around 3 hours. Because combined expertise and combined approaches make that possible. The angle of the sessions are about actively releasing more effectively the causes. Which could have taken hundreds of hours to talk through Hypnotherapy and associated approaches can release conflicts in very short time because the are targeted and efficient. The suggestions build great strength and would say rapport with the individuals unconscious mind. Therapists were institutions. They were famous for their name and their approaches, and still today though they were few and far between in these times when in the modern age though quality and efficacy varies between individuals.

The History and story of psychology comes from here into two branches, behaviorism and the science of suggestion such that they can coexist.

You will find the science of suggestion and behavior and thought correction on a conscious level at the same time as an unconscious level are a very potent formula. You will find inlaid in the book all three, the power of linguistic suggestion, hypnosis and relaxation and also perspective changing approaches. So the founding principles of behaviorism and the founding principles of advanced hypnosis techniques are included on a very subtle level.

The knowledge and learning is there for you to remember and self correct whereby the deeply embedded suggestion is to work subtly under the surface and engage many new and supportive choices.

Moving through time the development of behaviorism took hold over hypnosis especially in the minds of the common world. The mystical power of hypnosis some times incite fear of control which people had experiences to too many times. As wars across lands developed and the holocaust ensued the mass control of people deterred the supportive powers of mesmerism and the forces of great power established a firm fear in the minds of people as to the potency of suggestion. Sometimes when something has power to awaken there is great responsibility and it should always be used with integrity. Within the fears of the minds of people it appears that the fears pushed through different directions, now people are awakening to the potency being of an acceptable format. That Hypnosis and the power of suggestion is once again a helpful force.

The establishment behaviourism lines, including Pavlov and stimulus response pattern, they are all a potent form of suggestion and potent form of suggestion repetition and behavior change. Changing of neurological pathways to increase the potency of positive change within the nervous system and the fundamental changes to be experienced in life. Whether by increasing pain threshold or to act when necessary. In the 1900 Hypnosis began to build once more. In America Clarke Hull and learning and behaviour and internal drive theory based on needs and activating survival. Though of my most loved and pronounced hypnotherapists are George Estabrook's and Milton Erikson. Milton Erikson whos approaches ethos and methods move me in so many ways. Sadly he died in 1980, but he moved forward the works of Hull and is absolutely fascinating. Erikson would use story, much like you will when you are reading to your children he used metaphor and suggestion. The mind being symbolic Erikson would use the metaphor to make changed a very very deep but unseen level working with Ernest Rossi the psychobiology of mind body healing –Using suggestion to induce physiological healing such as healing the physical body using pendulums and ideo motor signals to incite healing. The potency of these aspects is within this book. To affect expediated healing post partum is simply down to the direction of your attention and the belief about what is possible. After a caesarean with my daughter I was discharged from hospital within 24 hours, usually you are retained for roughly 2 - 3 days minimum. Your body heals at an extraordinary rate when you are without complication and you ask it too. I was hanging washing out within 7 days. Hanging washing out … if you can imagine the muscles it uses to lift and stand and hang after a 9 month pregnancy and caesarean section surgery this is notable because it wasn't uncomfortable nor was there a risk to health or healing. The healing had progressed sufficiently in such a small space in time for that to be possible otherwise my body would have given me pain to stop me; You can do this too. Purely with your intentions. Reducing the risk of complication by intending smooth passage.

The intention was expediated healing. That every moment my body was healing new cells new strong connections cells healing, cool and calmness to the wound while I sleep while. I wake while a move walk speak sit always healing always restoring the energy in my body.

Because the would was healing every breath every moment healing for me and healing for baby something so simple as an intention through the intention was potent because of the belief that underlaid it that the body will heal and effectively and efficiently as possible. Is a deeply embedded belief of this kind can make waves of healing so great that the healing time is reduced dramatically. The pure intention of accelerated healing is often enough to actually affect it. So there are many many ways you can effectively use hypnotherapy to move forward in your life and to birth your baby with confidence and ease.

How will it feel when you know it has worked - I get asked this allot.

You won't. You won't have a comparison. A before and after. Because you have changed.

It is that subtle. You will just know.

You will have a hue. So go with the hue. And you will just change.

People often ask does it really work, The answer, does what work. The hypnotherapy works always. Does your mind not, work in making it work. That is debateable. The question, presupposes that it coud not work, it always works at some level. It can't not. When actually you are just making space for you to listen change and flourish.

And quite often you don't know unless you do it. And you don't know when you have, changed. Because it is that good. You can feel different. You can feel good. It isn't the worries that are keeping you alive, you just flow in different ways. Look different, you feel different, and you don't know why. You don't have to take it apart, question it, you can just feel good. And have a sense of intactness.

And the beauty of that is that the experience is different for everyone. The same reports, that they were calm and confident and it's as if time stopped and everything was easier, they felt so in control.

But each interpretation is different because everyone has different concerns to smooth through, and to overcome. The consistent repeated response is it works and feels good.

It is similar mentality to recent times a runner, had not tracked the milage but they had a place in mind they just run. Each step after the next. Preferably with music. A time in mind, occasional time check but it is another form of hypnosis.

It goes against so much of the goal setting last step focused thinking. Were programmed to keep thinking, checking in comparing where are you now etc, moving toward the next thing the next thing the next thing. That has a time and a place and a value but not in this context. When youre on a run, or birthing a baby they are timeless times. Though intensively timed. It iss like child birth once it starts you are in it. 100 percent once your run starts you are in it 100 percent until it ends.

But it works. It's the acceptance that that delusion is ok. That you can be that focused for that time in that bubble and that that is ok. They have the end in their heart. Rather than their mind. They just keep running. Have you ever seen Forest Gump when he just runs … it is something like that but with less beard.

So what is Hypnosis really, whats the science, show me the proof that's it's a something rather than a nothing. Here is the science building for the evidence lovers.

Have you heard of brain waves, the cyclic resonance of your mental activity reflected as electrical pusles registering in the brain.

These measure at a millionth of a volt. And there are 5 main frequencies registered in the human brain

They are Oscillations Measurements of the speed of Oscillation using a electroencephalology EEG. The five main brain activity frequencies are recognized as. The measurements are defined as hertz or cycles per second, ie, how many cycles of that wave from per second

Gamma: characteristics of this resonance are Problem solving and concentration – 30 hz or above

Beta : characteristics of this resonance are awake and alert – conversational.

14 – 30 hz

Alpha 7.5 – 14 Hz characteristics of this resonance are Relaxed waking state such as watching TV

Theta 4- 7.5 characteristics of this resonance are Asleep yet aware Suggestive capacity is great.

Delta 0.5 – 4 hz - characteristics of this resonance are Deep somnambulistic relaxation as if in a deep sleep.

These aren't measured in hypnosis but you can hear an actual real life scientific evidence that the frequency of your mental (brain) activity changes and that can be induced and influenced by relaxation.

The waves are impulses which could represent thoughts.

Calming thoughts calming mind calming waves of activity.

Therefore relaxation plus helpful language listened to gives way to unconscious change.

Im always wary of what people say around sleeping people. People under anesthesia.

And the more doctors and medical practitioners who learn how to communicate with the influence of helpful suggestions when they speak, the better.

You can innoculate yourself to accept helpful meanings from your medical practitioners words, so that you will always be accepting of the most helpful life enhancing elements of your wording.

For example.

People remember on a level everything that is said around them so always speak with intentions and kindness. Say it the way you want it. Hear it the way you want it. (but also hear what is said)

The levels of hypnosis

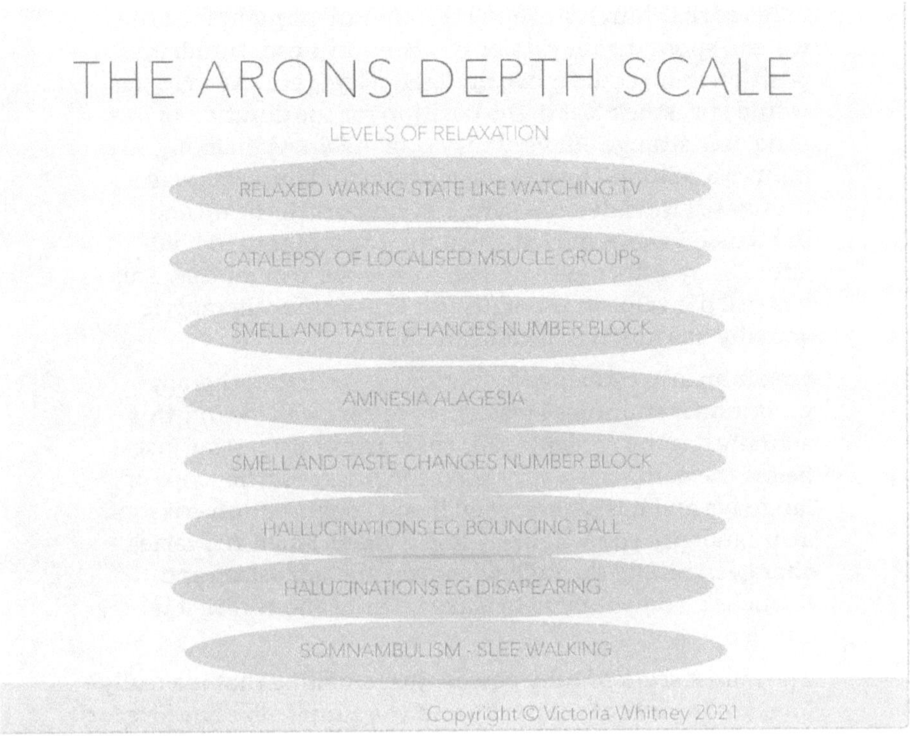

THE ARONS DEPTH SCALE

LEVELS OF RELAXATION

RELAXED WAKING STATE LIKE WATCHING TV

CATALEPSY OF LOCALISED MSUCLE GROUPS

SMELL AND TASTE CHANGES NUMBER BLOCK

AMNESIA ALAGESIA

SMELL AND TASTE CHANGES NUMBER BLOCK

HALLUCINATIONS EG BOUNCING BALL

HALUCINATIONS EG DISAPEARING

SOMNAMBULISM - SLEE WALKING

There are various levels to the state of relaxation induced by hypnotic guide hypnosis, levels of relaxation we experience most of them through the course of a day when we are relaxing sitting watching TV looking at the ocean, we do them from time to time.

One relaxation such as staring at the TV and tuning out. Just distraction, form thought so youre fixated on the tv and drift away in your consciousness

Two, Catalepsy of isolated muscle groups when you are distracted and you realize you are holding something, you are eating your toast and you are talking to someone, then you realize your arm has been in mid air holding the toast for a period of time.

The same with a mobile phone it is there in your hand you become Muscle groups here its held in mid air.

I did this at my child's christmas play recently. While I was holding the camera above my head high enough to take a video of the church stage, All through silent night my arms were in spontaneous catalepsy above my head. Numb in position as if I could move my head wiggle etc and my arms would stay stuck fast in the position for the duration of the song. It is strange but very very cool. Again when fixing a light to a ceiling. The mental effort to hold my arms was immense I intended my arms just support the beam and the tension was removed. Turning into strength to hold effortlessly. Effortless and doesn't tire the arm mucles. This has real life value. It is not just for show or for therapy. It actually has functional value in life.

I teach an arm catalepsy induction on the hypnotherapy practitioner trainings I teach here in cornwall uk and this actually has the students talk their arms into resting just below the chin. It is a very good convincer for the scope of language and it is potency and if you google Milton erikson arm catalepsy you will likely find a video. Smell and taste changes, sniffing the milk when you are half asleep and it smells ok only for you to wake up fully and realize it is curdled.

The purest scent of baby powder just smelling that is a really lovely reminder of the purity and the simplicity of he love for baby on those days when youre tired and you've had no sleep the night feeds are long and it is all there up in you. Breathe in the simplicity.

Breathe it in... scent of a baby, it wakes you up to the now of perfection rather than the thoughts of imperfection.

Both can be a state of hypnosis or trance we can be entranced on the what is not right or entranced into the whatever you need to be entranced by to make it right or you can be entranced. Into the lucidity of aliveness that is the best one.

Next levels of hypnosis, using Hallucinations, imagining each contraction as a bouncing ball each bounce bring you close to birthing your baby and having the pain easily subside. Visualising the bouncing ball in your minds eye. IS SO POWERFULL When you are contracting the rhythm of those contractions literally become the bouncing ball. And the energy of the bounce neutralises the sensation of the discomfort you would experience within had you not the hallucination, the visualisation of the bouncing ball to accompany the rhythm of the contraction.

The pain easily subside the pain easily subside because each
contraction brings you close to birthing your baby and
each bounce brings more comfort on the other side of the
contraction.

Then somnambulism the totally comatose feeling as if asleep.

Prioritising calming your mental activity reducing the
activity of your mind so you can tune out of external
stimulus and into you tunning into your inner mind tuning
into your body tunning into you.

Dissolving the distraction so you can go inside and create
build a place for complete faith safety trust and security that
brings you love and self acceptance. And the environment to
cultivate that which you want. That which you did not believe
possible until you thought .. what if...

So you can have the hue you can experience the hue and
the glow and the great shift in your perceptions beginning
to grow more coherent more merged and more within the
oneness.

It brings the sense of wholeness and connection between you
and baby between you and your body and between you and
the belief that you are capable you are calm you are balanced
and you are centred.

Uncovering your natural ability to birth your baby with ease
birth you baby with confidence and birth your baby with the
strength of you full consciousness working with you. Your
full womanhood working with you in a gentle and subtle way.

Bridging the space between you and your experience of
childbirth being anything other than what you would hope
for and what you are capable of determining.

When the space withing you for birth is established your body
moves and works with you as one.

The space within you for the birth is one and the hue is
within you you have a sense of effortlessness and grace and of
complete self assurance even when challenges are faced you
have the sense of one ness with yourself

Specifically for child birth most challenging situations this
teaches you to stop,

Slow down and stay present in the moment, without even

thinking because that's wat you are naturally aligned to do.

Ultimately you were born to do this … you were born to read this and to discover this about you. Your brain what it is doing and how you can use it in another way to the way you already learned.

The power of intention the power of suggestion and the power of a turn on a perspective is immeasurable. But measurable as a frequency and resonance

Below is relaxation session transcript – if you look at the references page you will find links to the recorded audios available to purchase for a nominal admin fee. But here is the thing. I can only sell up to 1000 copies per year. Which is strict due to the trademark and copyright permissions. So get there first as they are definitely worth it.

Relaxation session...

Simply close you eyes and let everything else fade away in importance

I want you to think of the word relax ......

Think about how it has two syllables

Re lax......

As you breathe in think

Re to yourself

And as you breathe out

Think lax

Don't let your mind wander away for repeating the word relax

When you breathe out try to let go of any tension in your body

Focus on those muscles, which may have been holding some tension

Every time you breathe out lax the out breath is the one to focus on

The in breath takes care of itself

Think re on each breath in and lax on each breath out

Imagine those out breaths

Are being blown into a big balloon all of your tensions being expelled from your body and being blown into that big balloon

The balloon being filled up with air and when it is full imagine it floating away

And as it floats away the balloon carries away all of those tensions

And you are feeling completely in control

Allow your hands to rest comfortably on top of your legs wherever they feel most comfortable

Now as you relax more and let it go more and more

You can allow every muscle in your body to relax

Every cell every nerve every fiber in your body relaxing

Now picture in your mind a candle this candle can be any color you with it to be

The color you have chosen for your candle is a color you unconscious mind knows relaxes you and calms your mind

Calms you and relaxes your mind. It is your color of calm

Now focus on you the color of the flame of the candle

See how amazing the colors within the flame are

You may see red, blue yellow purple white

And maybe another color

And as you see the colors within the flame you relax more and more

And go deeper

And as you enjoy these heavy and relaxed feelings deeply relaxed feelings

These feelings of being in control.

Now focus on the wax body of your candle

Now see the first trickle of melting wax begin to move down the wax

Now see the melting wax touch the candleholder and merge with it to become part of the candleholder

You become more and more relaxed

Feeling safe and comfortable

Now imagine that you re that candle

A candle of total relaxation

And as you picture it a particular muscle in your body melts away it is tension allowing you to relax more and more completely

Picture whatever you are sitting or lying on as a candle holder and that youre becoming yourself a candle of relaxation

Feel yourself melting into the experience of childbirth

Your body simply melting into the task of doing what it knows how to do

You are feeling calm confident and in control

And because you are feeling calm confident and in control your body follows your mind as your mind relaxes

And your mind follows your body

As our body relaxes

Your baby too is feeling calm trusting the experience and trusting you

Notice how you have to been aware of any sensations of the area of your body that your hands have been resting on until you choose to switch your awareness there

In the same way you can choose which sensations which sensations to be aware of or to focus on during you labor

Now I will count form 1 up to 10

And as I count I want you to imagine you are seeing your baby for the first time

1, 2, 3,

Notice how much more in control you are feeling

Four

Five

Calm confident and in control

6

7

8

Becoming more aware of the room now

9

Because you choose to become aware of the room

10

In your own time open your eyes and become aware of the room you are in.

Dont just try it. Do it. Use it. It will make a difference.

Recap, so now you are pregnant. You know why, You definitely know how, and you have an understanding how hypnosis for child birth works, you have experienced it. Now to learn about your body.

CHAPTER 3

Your Body

"Everything grows rounder and wider and weirder, and
I sit here in the middle of it all and wonder who in the
world you will turn out to be." — Carrie Fisher

Your body in fascinating detail

It's a miracle.

Living breathing walking talking miracle

We don't celebrate it enough - we don't
celebrate our bodies enough

They wake up our heart beats, we breathe we ourselves were formed from a single egg and grew in our mothers womb. You are growing a miracle. You are growing a small human. Every time we scuff our body it heals. There is a predisposed ability for your body to heal and re grow. And the ability to release the trauma of the injury . Our bones heal and re grow. Your body is a constantly repairing and replenishing itself all of the time and in in pregnancy it is magnified and directed. What makes the most difference is the emotional resonance you are carrying within you to expediate healing and to experience healing. What your body is capable of is unknown until it is tested. People do iron man, run 100 mile ultra marathons and that is just one single thing in the degree of endurance human body is capable of.

When you think about the potential your body has,
childbirth isn't such a great expectation.

To make childbirth comfortable and to guide and push your baby through the birth canal as comfortable and efficiently as possible isn't a huge expectation. The greatest task is to maintain your mental focus and clarity and composure to allow for the body to progress within the purpose focused solely on one task to birth your baby.

The greatest task is to allow your body to do what it can do, to trust you body and to have faith in it is ability to birth your baby. This you will learn is to centre and focus your attention of the miracle of your body and develop the faith in it is ability to birth baby and for this task hypnosis was perfectly developed, perfectly matched and perfectly delivered.

Your body has manufactured an entire life support system for your baby and you as it's host. You have a unique life support system within you a life growth system. Fully engineered and perfected by you, without thought. Without conscious design. Or without intervention. You just are it.

You just are.

Every day it gets up and every day we breathe every day our cells just seem to renew and regenerate every day our body just works If you have a cut it heals. If you are really hopeful, without scar. Yes sometimes it has a moment of weakness when something in our internal system isn't working, and requires repair. And some intervention. But on the whole your body is a miracle, a living breathing walking talking miracle.

Every aspect of your body is perfectly designed to fulfil a role to keep you alive and do something.

The body in more detail, firstly Your Uterus is amazing. It is so intricately constructed, to both harness and to provide life support to your baby that it is truly amazing.

The placenta the very cellular growth daily formation and the role your uterus fulfils is incredible. What your uterus can achieve over this 40 weeks is beyond comprehension, and if your uterus can from this actually grow it. Imagine what the rest of your body and mind are capable when they work in harmony. With your natural rhythm, and your natural sense of what you do really desire and what you were born to do.

From one egg and a sperm cell it creates a home for a 40 week journey of cellular construction form an egg to a human. A secure unit of absolutely everything is fulfilled and converted into life support for your baby so it can grow and it can develop and it can become and it can not just live but thrive. Your uterus and placenta provides the actual moment by moment conversion and calculation of everything that baby needs. In the external environment how many machines does it take to keep that role fulfilled when your body can do it all within itself. The intelligence of your body is phenomenal. You do that. Without even thinking. When you are unconsciously weighing out milk formula ... and how much science it takes to engineer to formula we buy, your body does that. Just by its ultra design, it naturally adjust the formulaic components of your milk perfectly for baby. You are that in tune. . It does this in Utero for the full 9 months. Everything your baby needs is provided. Just like for you when you were in the womb. Everything was provided for you not necessarily by your mother but by the consciousness that was her body. Which you can assume as a belief that everything will be provided unto you. Just like when you are a child, you grew your body knew how. Just like you. As your consciousness can provide for you and your baby everything you need to not just survive but also thrive. Because you can do this for you too unconsciously. Meaning believe there is something more than we can control, so have a sense of humility in awe of what your body is doing capable of. Brushing our ego to one side

Your uterus - OMG - is amazing – is not a sentence I ever, ever thought I would hear myself saying on any day in any way. But it is true. As far as organs go our hearts beat and our lungs breathe but actually your uterus grows small human, along with the support and cohesion of our other organs. It grows an actual person. Immaculately and that's what it is programmed to do to create a life support system for baby. Of course the egg and sperm have their role and the foetus knows how to grow, just like seeds when you plant them.

With that known idea that childbirth without fear is pre programmed into your body to just do it. As long as we stay out of the way. Breathe, relax, and work with our body it can do it. Your uterus has never been so sexy. Just the dimensions and facts...

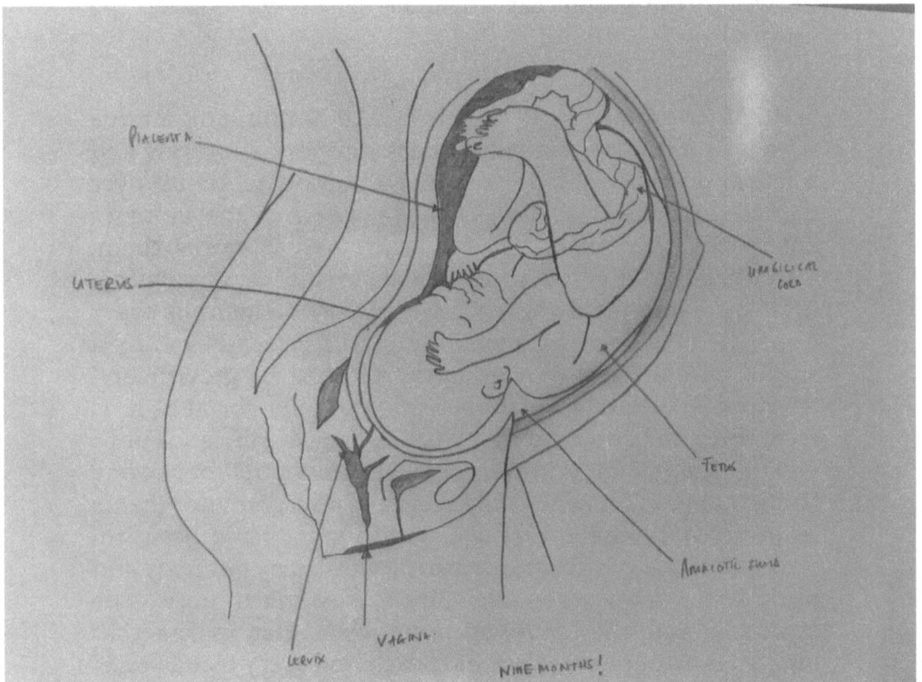

14 inch muscular purse ½ inch think

16 weeks 2 inches below navel

23 weeks its peak is at navel 7 months 2- 3 inches above the navel.

38 weeks highest point in abdomen

40 weeks drops 2 inches as head engages and water reduces.

12 weeks: most organs are formed.

14 weeks: doctors can tell the sex of the foetus.

16 to 20 weeks: you may be able to feel movement.

24 weeks: the foetus has a chance of survival outside the uterus.

Perhaps the most selfless act of the unthinking uterus without ego it makes sure that baby develops as quickly and safely as possible so that it can thrive without it. In just over half its predicted use time. Just 24 weeks in the event of emergency there it is. It has skills and it works them. Throughout that whole time. Living. breathing. Circulating. Giving life and taking waste a way. Every moment of every day. The uterus grows a small human from and egg and a sperm and sustains it through 9 months of growth and development into a small person. Perfectly formed. It is something to behold, to many it has little significance until you think about it it is just a womb. It's an example of just one thing that goes on behind the scenes of our ignorance that is so perfectly innately ordained within us. Such a beautiful example of the structure that can be weaved by our body and mind in harmony when in reality it is so much more. The structure and the interwoven network that makes that happen is astounding. Each fibre each and every blood vessel uniquely defined and designed to not just withstand but also withhold the growth of a foetus through 9 months. The growth of each and every skin cell every organ and every single cell of baby that forms into its perfectly organized human self. The unique infrastructure beautifully supports sustains and grows life. And it is within you. Every Single cell of their body and every aspect of the self is designed to make this life and when they are signed with the essence of themselves and the miracle of the simplicity that makes their body makes their heart beat they will always succeed as a parent because it is not static, it is transient and transitory moves and grows just like the womb. Imagine your world can change in just the same way. Changed it's structure to accommodate the growing foetus, so do our minds our bodies our souls expand our lives just like a mirror image of the growth inside. Your abilty to make really strong changes is also greater. You think purer in pregnancy you put what is best for you into your body by reducing alcohol and anything that is not recommended, You are really in the best shape of your life chemically, while you are pregnant so in the same token you will be believing cleaner, and your body will function better as a vehicle for making what you want into life. There is a different form of respect you have for your body, your mind and your purpose is to protect grow and nurture. When you support your body and mind in making the environment in your body that is harmonious with your and babies best health your life will turn to support you. Even if you don't fully believe it. It will tend to. Life accommodates us when we trust it.   Trust is quiet. It is that sense of composure, not a feeling, it is a togetherness, intactness. What's more we aren't even done with you womb yet. There is more. They do come with challenge practical and functional but with the incredible medical care available they can each be over come one by one. There is always a way. It may not be easy but there is always a way It's a 14 inch muscular organ With both latitudinal and longitudinal muscles. Weaved like the global geographic coordinate system. Right inside you. A mirror of the globe, the world. They weave together to its Inner layer of figure of 8 mesh fibres which all contract in harmony through contraction in labour, and hold stable while baby is growing through the three trimesters. That's 10 whole months. It provides blood and takes away waste product alongside the placenta from its own exertion in growth on a constant level until the babies birth. It's a cycle of growth and a life in and of itself. With its own purpose which is very profound and very beautiful. It is a work of art. The diagrams are clearly organic. They are owned by Victoria so the copyright privileges attached are indisputable.

The uterus with the muscle layers defined.

The Uterus - Outer layer longitudinal fibres.

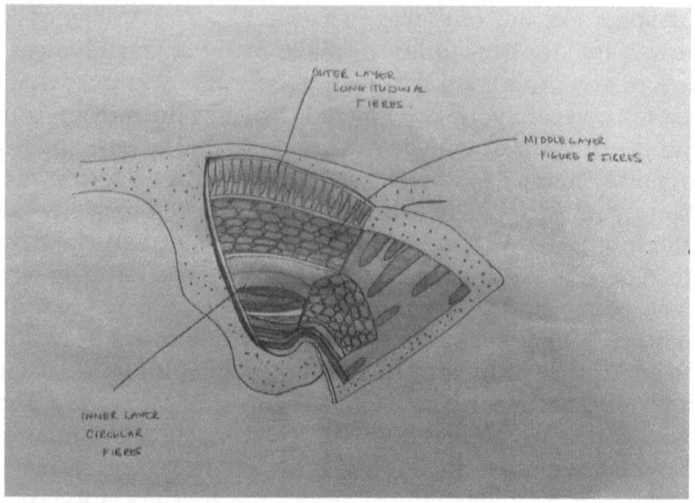

Middle layer Figure 8 fibres
Inner layer circular fibres. They grow they weave they encircle they encapsulate baby in a space of you and that is so beautiful. Spherical and ellipsoidal. They move in a Mexican wave to enable baby to birth through the birth canal .. rhythmic muscle stimulations and sensations as waves of electrical nerve impulses cause contraction. Literally like a wave of movement moving through your body. Something so daunting and so intense conceptually could overtake you, as if it is stronger than you. It is but it is not, you work with it, contractions are built up to sound terrifying, but they are a process of Rhythm and movement, which you can work with and through. The main role of your consciousness is to move with the relaxation of your body will allow it to do what it is naturally designed to do. The only temptation is to worry and to fear. This is the least effective and last thing you should do. The body is weaved by an artist who demanded perfection at its greatest Our thinking and fear just gets in the way. Intricately weaved web of fine musculature to cradle baby through its term and then wave by wave breath by breath, electrical nerve impulse to impulse causing the body to contract that is the birth journey.

It is a work of art in it's form. A thing so great and so magnificent that to simplify it by the word womb is futile its immaculate infrastructure is so defined, its resonance is of absolute purity and beauty as it cradles small life, nourishes and in its later stages of term births it into life.

One of the least known but the absolute coolest reflex in the human body is the Fergusson Reflex. Babies desire to breathe is one trigger in the process of birth. It stimulates the Fergusson reflex which in turn, combined with babies head pressing onto the cervix, begins contractions and starts the process of birth. A self-sustaining sequence and cycle of uterine contractions - A neuro endocrine reflex. Impressive. And further supports. The notion that with a state of fearlessness and complete centredness, calm relaxation in the hue, in the moment and journey of childbirth you are able to, fully able to birth baby with ease. Your body can do it without your consciousness. So what are you going to choose to do with your consciousness other than support you body in doing what it was created and designed to do by trusting it and loving it and believing in it, and learning to work with your body staying calm confident and in control. If all you had to do was to stay calm and work with the movements of your body. It's so simple, yet so profound. There are examples mostly in the US where women in coma have birthed babies naturally - they have been found to be pregnant and then spontaneously birthed healthy babies. The principle and the case in point is that the body can do this. Without thinking. So when your thoughts are supportive and faith loaded. There is a greater supportive force within you. Using the audio downloads and scripts your mind will induce your mind scattered thoughts, the doubts and the unknowns to subside, they will calm, and you will have the hue. By alleviating the fears you are redirecting your energy through your body to work with you. The fears and the doubts the permeating insidious influence of worry will roll of your teflon coating. The anxieties will wash away, Because they will have nothing to stick to. You will unconsciously without effort experience the building of a force field. Like the uterus for baby but for you and your belief structure, the only difference you can retain this one after birth and it will just get stronger. But it can fully support you. Fully sustain you as you feed it you nourish it. You can fully focus and concentrate on being pregnant and birthing baby. Birthing baby. Is what your body is designed to do even without thought. It's a reflex. So the only things that sits between you and birthing baby with ease are fears, tensions and the fixation of your attention. The methods in birthing babies elevate the worries fears and give you ways to channel your attention to assist you in progressing the discomfort and the energy of labour in a way that is beneficial. It is working with your body. Knowing how your body works and also knowing how your energy and attention can all form together to support that is new and great. That being true the only essence that makes labour less easy other than a physical anomaly is fear and tension. According to Hopkins Medical Research Unit at John Hopkins Hospital Only 8% of pregnancies have physical complications. [2] The unknown truth is that Child Birth is a reflex. As you draw closer to your due date, I explain more for this later. Oxytocin is long known as the love drug, A relaxant and present in both intimacy and birth. Oxytocin production is triggered when babies head pushes upon the cervix the production of oxytocin initiates and the reflex begins. The intensity of the oxytocin receptors in your womb increase by 200 fold. This means that your uterus is perfectly primed to react to this hormone. Imagine this was caffeine - and the receptors increased in equal measure. Just imagine. A 200 fold magnification of your morning coffee. This is something I would not want to see but if you can appreciate the relative difference and the supportive influence of the immaculate design of your body and the birthing process. Then you have a lot of natural anaesthesia already circulating your nervous system encouraging a sense of relaxation and euphoria. Most people don't know this.

You increased the receptors for maximum uptake and maximum effectiveness of the purpose of the hormones. That's a 200 percent magnification to alleviate the tension and expand the muscle fibres and lessen the sensation of the expansion, as your baby moves through the birth canal the relaxation and expansion of the fibres all enhanced by the chemical of oxytocin enriching every cell fibre to ease the sensations of expansion and discomfort.

Your body is a symphony, there is an internal an orchestra all the instruments playing in symphony and that symphony is you. That's what stimulated the production of oxytocin the contraction of muscles through relaxation of certain muscle groups. Ironically it's the relaxation induced by the love drug oxytocin that brings about the contraction of the muscles. That progresses the interaction between the uterine wall and the contractions. It desensitises the parameter walls so that you can reduce the discomfort to allow for the expansion.

That progresses the contraction and relaxation of the uterine wall in a Mexican wave form to bring about the progression of the baby through the birth canal.

They come in all shapes and sizes each one unique in it's form and each one perfect in and of itself. Typically, it presents as an upside down pear shape. They can be heart shape or variations in between. Practically and functionally, all shapes and sizes. Very beautifully interwoven composure of longitudinal and latitudinal muscles. Each forming a web a web of support that weaves its strength around your baby ensuring 10 months of growth and development. Strengthening with each fibre relaces itself and grows stronger moment by moment to accommodate your babies growing body. Looking back to the Fergusson reflex and your body. The physical process of birth of baby as a reflex. The one most powerful influence you have is to centralise your mind centralise your thoughts and bring about the fixation of attention. On you being calm, confident and in control of your mind, this is mirrored in your body so that your body can birth baby as was intended by design. Trust your body to birth baby.

Until now ... the potential to reduce the length of your labour by simply moving thoughts, contradictions out of the way. Turning Fear into faith moving the focus of your attention from not knowing what is happening to what is happening in your body. To expedite the natural laboric flow. The word laboric doesn't exist in the English directory but as a process or a name to describe a sequence or the entity of a process. The word as a name laboric even means "You appear strong and powerful. You have an impressive personality and can influence and even intimidate through sheer force" The sheer force of natural birth interesting huh. It's a much more effective turn on the phrase labour which has an embrandmnet of arduous process into a natural flowing sequence. I speak this way though I have experienced full labour. It does require effort and focus and concentration and relaxation and birthing a baby is not quite as effort less as a sneeze. But it is easier when you know what is happening it is easier when you move with our body and it is easier when you are aware your body is moving you. When you can grasp that your body is working with you more than your mind then you have the space to make your mind move with the education that shows your mind and body how to work together, in a way that is much more effective. Efficient. In learning a sport you actually have to relay so many new proprioceptive alignments in your muscles and brain and cohere the two, here it is different with childbirth it is all seeded unconsciously. Your body knows what to do. Working with the mind body connection. Which in some ways is the backwards how. At this point the presupposition that labour should be arduous is not helpful. So we can instead assume that it can be a pleasurable experience.

The Mind body connection

A paradigm simplifies the interaction which will define your greatest life choices. Which ever way around you roll the dice of the order and organization that always work effectively for you. You can use the chain of interaction in any of the three routes. For example. This book is using your mind by being in your environment to influence your body and it works by using your thoughts to change the resonance of your body and influence your environment by making choices differently to how you would have made the before because you are strengthened in resolve and have more information, you are more educated so less swayed by the environment and therefore have more traction to influence the environment. This is empowerment. You are more able to move the situation to your advantage and favour because you have a stronger foothold of knowledge than you did before. That becomes a bed of faith, your fall back. You choose the way your mind influences you body and you choose how your environment works for you the interaction between all 3 makes movement more comfortable.

THE MIND BODY CONNECTION

Mind

Body   Environment

Mind

There is known many known medical professionals Doctors who have identified a deep connection between our thoughts and our bodies health, and our experience of life. The thought leaders in this spectrum include. Louise Hay, Candace Pert who looked into the emotional effect on molecular structures, Bruce Lipton in the biology of belief who has the essence of the interaction between thoughts and cells being. Greg Braden and the Divine matrix the interconnectedness for the basic principle thoughts creating things amplified by feeling.

Hidden messages of water massaru emoto - a book which brought to life actual pictorial evidence the influence on intention words onto the frozen water.

The words love and gratitude made the crystalline structure very beautiful intricately woven crystalline structures actual symmetrical form so beautiful. Clean and crisp and organised, elegant and refined. And words hate and fear made the crystalline structures deformed and mutated, harsh and asymmetrical

This being true then the resonance of our cellular structure being water is heavily influenced by the components of communication what occurs within and around us what we say what we do, what we think. We literally absorb it from the environment around us. Until like you are now. As your beliefs turn and strengthens so you are less influenced by the environmental influences, what begins to resonate with you as you are moving forward.

Literally absorb like a sponge until you know that you can choose whether it's a useful addition or not, so you can build a strength in awareness you choose to filter what you see and hear consciously. So like when baby is 8 weeks old you might choose to inoculate it from certain illnesses. You can inoculate yourself from unhelpful influences by building resistance. By building different beliefs, intentions and forging different paths. Consider supportive beliefs as the antibodies. Built to strengthen and secure your immunity to ... whatever is the unhelpful influence.

Instead what you will do is strengthen your core beliefs just like your body building muscle. You will strengthen your beliefs and your bubble so that you will be teflon coated. You will just know what is right for you and that is what birthing babies as a journey enables you to do. Almost effortless because as your beliefs strengthen the hue strengthens, like a layer of support around you invisibly and within you incubating you, as well as inoculating you from the perceptions that would lower your perceptions and incite fear.

Belief by osmosis is a given in life, it happens, thought now you are aware you can choose. And as you're building your Hue, it will work for you. The thoughts we have are instruction to our cells the words we use are instructions to our cells It influences our resonance so listening to birthing babies and absorbing this book will only add helpful influences supportive layer of consciousness that can become you without effort. That is the value. A high return on investment of time. Because it can't not become you in some way. It moves you. Into being, something more capable more competent and stronger to the extent you believe it will so go all in. And to find value for you within you so long as you allow it to. Ensure we are resonating with a frequency within that is in alignment with birthing baby comfortably that means allowing the reflexes to be effective that means allowing our reflexes to be effective by conspiritus thoughts to the contrary being evacuated and being overwritten by more supportive ideas and resonance. With each thought that changes a new resonance begins and that is the value of your mind and its ability to transition. Every day your body is making new cells. When you imagine the influence. Instead what you will do is strengthen your core beliefs just like your body building Muscle. You will strengthen your beliefs and your bubble so that it will actually like water of a ducks back rather then sifting through them. You will just know what is right for you and that is what birthing babies as a journey enables you to do. Almost effortless because as your beliefs strengthen the hue strengthens, like a layer of support around you invisibly and within you incubating you, as well as inoculating you from the perceptions that would lower your perceptions and incite fear. When you imagine the influence what was a threat and what was not. Now our sensory environment contains so much which we believe is good for us but is actually not always the case. Our nervous system is confused by the amount of stimulation that is available to us. Your chemical load is different now. The chemical load comprises many many stimulus from our environment be it digital be it consequential from interactions in our every day life. So tuning out of the noise and into your body.

To allow the birth process to progress birth and allow for the opening of the cervix, contraction of the uterine muscles all led by babies desire to breath and the first kick response.

Your body is linked to your thoughts, so mind and body work in harmony.

Your environment : Includes, actions behaviours, and also physical complication such as breach positioning and placenta positioning these are idiosyncracies that can factor into birth planning and the process of birth however you can still control your experience of birth the process and the experience do not always define each other.

Environment includes professionals and decisions about birth planning. The places and spaces around you. What you put in your body.

The places you spend time - If you listen to fearful people you will experience fearful thoughts though if you listen to the feelings of being calm confident and in control. Then you will experience being calm confident and in control.

Example, fearful people, with dramatic stories of woe. Literally feeding your mind with stories of woe and risk this is what is nourishing your mind. Change that. Learn something different.

When you absorb what you read hear including this book and relaxation sessions it will inoculate you within into a bubble of your own strength of thought and belief so no matter what the environmental circumstances are, you are stronger within, to both manage the environment. Either change it or work with it or form a new plan. You will have their knowledge working within you for you. It Inoculates you without you even thinking. You build a confidence, once again it's the hue. The hue is for you and contains a strength and intactness. As you listen, as you live and as you learn it all comes together. It all becomes you and you become strong. That is the hue.

Here chapter by chapter form new solidifying beliefs. Covering all of these angles so you can evolve into a new level of mind body environment control and cohesion. It's not even about connection it is about a cohesion. Building your invisible strength.

You will have more coherence within the space of your mind and it's internal control even opposite of external challenge.

More thought and idea about the way your own body and mind and environment correlate and how they can all work in harmony for you and nurture each in turn to form a cohesive flow which works for you both through pregnancy birth and beyond.

Pain versus Discomfort

Pain and discomfort - The strangest paradox is that pain is amplified by the tension in your mind through to your body in a way that causes the neurological impulses in the body that create tension and in turn the tension then cause constriction which in turn causes pain.

So when you take it back to basics - The potential that you think pain into being to some degree. Is helpful because you can unthink it.

Not in its entirety, so you have mechanisms here that will enable you to reduce the sensation of pain reduce the sensation of pain. And the pain will become some sense of discomfort in a reduced form.

The reduction of the sensation of pain is brought about by the balancing of the sensations within your mind that transmits the signals though neurotransmitters alerting to movement and change therefore indicating an unknown and that something is different. When the signal causes tension this slows the progression of the fergusson reflexive impulses chemically be reducing the amount of oxytocin produced and increasing the amount of adrenaline and stress hormones such as cortisol which will inhibit the production and uptake of oxytocin and slow the progression of labour. It is a very clean conscience. When you reduce the fear. The experience is improved for both you and baby.

The Aim – The Three C's

THE THREE C'S

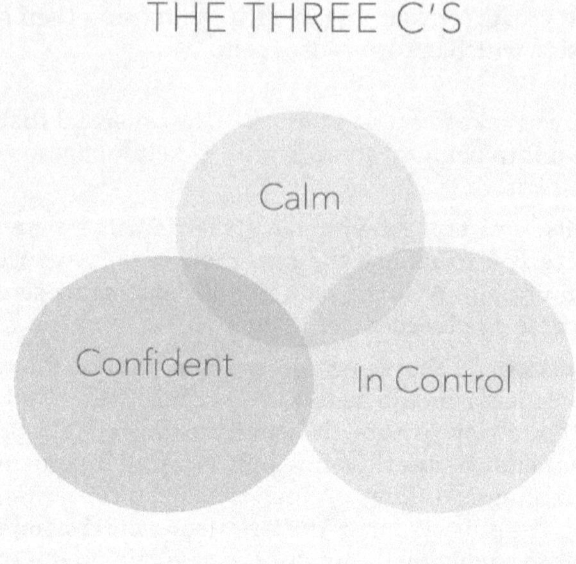

The role of the hormones

We have an autonomic nervous system which is a component of the peripheral nervous system regulating involuntary responses such as heart rate, blood pressure, respiration, digestion and circulation.

There are two branches of the Autonomic nervous system - sympathetic and parasympathetic.

Parasympathetic nervous system. Is heightened states of attention, wellbeing and flow of the attention and systems within your body circulating health and wellbeing and underpinning a greater sense of health and well being. Of type B behaviour. Attentive, forgiving and laid back, warm hands slow breath.

Sympathetic nervous arousal is the sense of type A behaviour stress state and the feeling of woundupness. Where there is less flow of circulatory system the heart beats faster and there is sense of general constriction. Cold hands. Fast breath.

One is greater tension and one has greater flow.

You can simplify it once more

Faith VS FEAR. Faith is born from fear and the two cannot coexist simultaneously in the human nervous system.

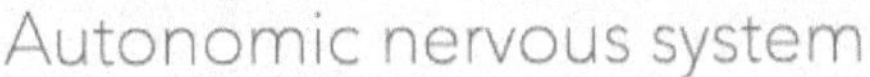

THE SCIENCE PART - THE ROLE OF HORMONES

Autonomic nervous system

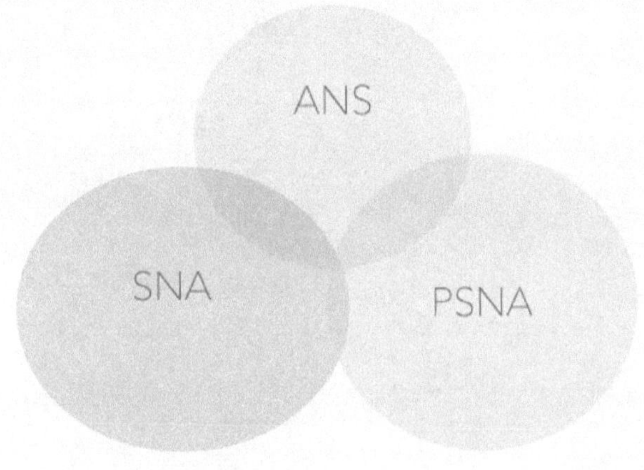

The fear tension pain paradigm is caused as above thinking the thoughts and sensation of pain into the body causing constriction.

The reverse of constriction is to alleviate the fears and bring within the sense of calm confidence and the application of helpful mechanisms of thought which will reduce the sensation of pain while keeping the functional purposes of pain as an instinctive response to the sensations of change within the body. Then you can be comfortably altered to action should the pain be a symptom requiring the attention of medical practitioners eg

If you experience cramping and bleeding it's important to

instinctively calmly seek and follow medical advice.

◆ ◆ ◆

THE SCIENCE PART - THE ROLE OF HORMONES

Pain paradigm

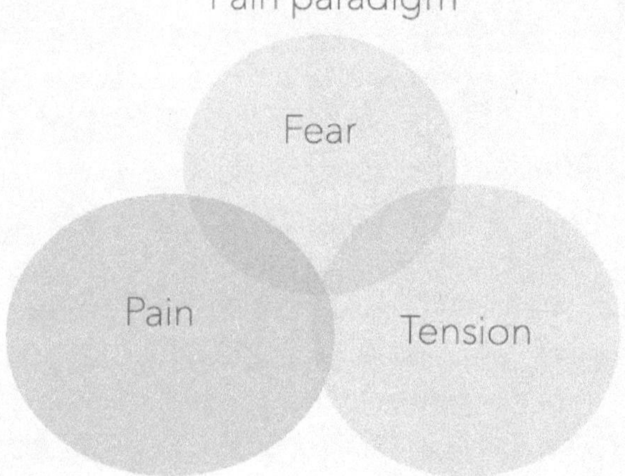

When the fear amplified the discomfort into pain causing tension. Alternated to calm. Realistically educated through this book into knowing your body knowing what hypnosis is knowing the chemistry turning fears into faith and then imagine how different your relationship with pain will actually be. Everyone has their own pain threshold. And it can change.

Your educated filters change the relationship you have with pain and the fears, and the experience of discomfort. That is caused the tension and caused the pain in the first place so you will by-product of reading this book alter your level of pain. And the more you work with the concepts the pain will be reduced. Does this mean you can't use pain medication.

Hell no.

It's just an addition. It's your choice. Some people do For various reasons, chemicals and baby, for their own strength everyone's birth choices are personal and there is a no judgement. It's your choice. This is just the space where you can define your own journey to use a phenomenal amount of your own personal attention to centre your mind and work with your body to birth baby.

THE SCIENCE PART - THE ROLE OF HORMONES

Reverse pain paradigm

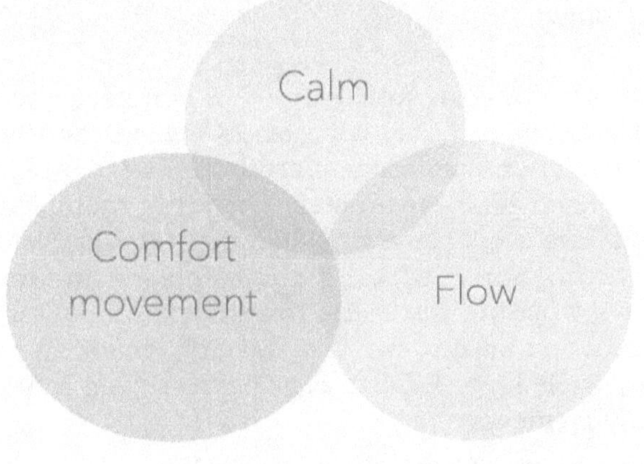

It's engaging, you are engaging your logical thinking educated brain with an innate truth which has not been introduced until now. Everything you need inside to be calm confident and in control is already within you. But now you are explaining how. The logic supports the calm, it's a win win that you can use anywhere in life. There are some limited statistics though I'm cautious regarding the pain medication reduction or medication free birth, bite your stick just get on with it and remain very much pro choice in the moment. Because every birth is different.

Dick Grantly Reed was a leading advocate of relaxation and child birth and his book child birth without fear is a very helpful and eye opening conceptual shift on child birth and the relationship to pain from the early 1900's. There are as we look at labour later on, other ways to manage pain and if you choose medication that's ok. Your birth your choice.

In case you questions, even though it is your choice. Personally did I - No. There wasn't time. I used gas and air for the last hour and a cocodamol tablet 5 hours before birth when I thought it was just movement. I was expecting immense pain, but it was just so subtle. Like cramps, but a little bit stronger.

Sometimes you have to work with what you have and that is what I did. My son was born at 38 plus 2 and was a footling breach (undiagnosed) Born in an ambulance just a mile from the hospital. Fortunately I had this. And the exact audios you have available. Even when there was challenging circumstance. I remained calm confident and in control. Would you – when you get there. You don't know how strong you are until you need to be. And this only builds and adds another invisible layer. Evidences as below so you can make your own judgements [3]

Bobart and Brown - The Efficacy of Medication

2002 72 mothers 36 had hypnotherapy sessions

Regional anaesthesia in the control group – 95% - Hypnosis group 38% (epidural)

Analgesia in the control group 75% - Hypnosis group 5.5 % (pethadine, cocodamol gas and air)

No analgesia or pre med –

In the control group 2.7% Hypnosis group 61%.

There is the evidence in one study, you can draw your own conclusions from this.

Other notifications of health. Apgar scores are an immediate measure of the physical condition of a newborn infant. It is obtained by adding points (2, 1, or 0) for heart rate, respiratory effort, muscle tone, response to stimulation, and skin coloration; a score of ten represents the best possible condition. This is an immediate assessment of your babies health and wellbeing. They do not predict mortality as they can improve very quickly.

If birth is long and arduous they can be lower. Or if there is a requirement for intervention they may be lower. As you can imagine. After a 20 hour working day you would be tired. If this 20 hour work day was graced with a resonance of rejuvenation and complete love and faith and fixation on absolute love, intactness and an internal faith, that everything good in you was working with you for you to achieve the days task you would likely feel less exhausted. As would baby as your passenger. There is a parallel between the induction of stress on the body and lower health. That is fact. Relaxation as an enhancement brought about by the relaxation and sense and strength of calm within the woman who births are sensical. Well being, being referred to baby and in turn every time you listen to a relaxation audio the greater health and well being that will prevail. Fears are transitory. There is a sensical truth. No matter how we reason out of it, no matter how we begin to embody the disquiet that is the opposition, the uprising and the denial of a latent truth. It isn't a statement of imposition of a belief, it is science. Saying that relaxation and the strength of fixation of attention on calm balance within the birthing woman brings greater health to the woman and the baby. That is sensical. That is truth and it is evident Birth Apgar scores higher when babies are born with hypnosis for child birth. It makes sense. Calm mother calm baby the physiological components laid out it makes sense chemically, physically and environmentally no matter how much intervention is required. It is still possible. Because the influence is on your experience. Your body your attitude, your perspective. So your focus changes and therefore yours and your babies experience of birth changes into something within your experience as something that you can control.

It's is suggested that babies have better infant apgar scores following hypnosis and a shorter stage 1 labour [4] Whether this is a proven fact or simply a theory makes little difference in reality. I have seen many times when there are no statistical significance of benefits of uses of therapies. Yet had I recorded their effectiveness by asserting the same principles that I do routinely and applied from my back dated experience of statistical significance from Psychology training many years ago, I would have likely found significance. The significance isn't that which is to provide a factual base for individuals to decide. There is a time when there is a requirement for this, but most often the actual faith that something is to effectively transition your thinking between the space of fear and faith is a leap. These leaps don't often have a basis of factual evidence because often it is too remarkable for us even to imagine as true. Faith is immeasurable.

If we did we would be forced to believe in something greater than ourselves which is a leap in and of itself. We are very much for proof, and empirical data. And sometimes to make something empirical sometimes limits it's potential expansion because it is so definitive. You can't measure the difference in someones eyes when they have cleared a lifelong problem with numbers. You can ask questions to empirically prove the difference. But to suggest that something does not work because it is not empirically tested can lead to ignorance of a great solution.

It is the change in peoples lives, health and the equivalent in life changes that is evidence enough. That is real and solid. And to them and that is why they return, that is why they continue because it works. Listen to one audio time after time and notice how things change.

It is the hue. It is invisible but remarkably visible and it brings such great strength and fortitude. That is what resonates within you through your birthing journey. The hue is what you make it. If you could make it what you wanted would you.

Looking through the whole perspectives you can sensically assemble that the calm confident and in control sensation when resonating through your body will resonate through to baby and baby will receive more oxygen and all of the benefits of reduced stress hormone through the transition from womb to life.

You can look at the medication angle – gas and air will have minimal influence on the baby, because the placenta is so good at breaking down toxins and protecting your baby from any harmful effects. Even some forms of Chemotherapy don't cross the placenta it is that well formed.

More statistics when hypnosis is present.

Rates of intervention 38/ 45 delivered spontaneously without need for intervention which includes venteuse, forceps and caesarean.

84 % higher than population as a whole.

Again more evidence.

Always remembering that you are in control of your mind. Your emotions and your body. How you live your body through breath and intention. It is possible to birth baby comfortably and more efficiently.

So the health benefits to you and baby are evident just by staying calm, confident and in control.

In short, you have the ability to maintain your equilibrium of calm, confidence and in control and now you know why. You are educated. The chemicals speak for themselves.

Your body is a miracle and when you see it through your educated eyes. Where the natural cycles come together in synergy, birth is easier. Have faith and confidence that you can birth a baby just the way you want. No matter what happens.

Another layer of truth built in the sensical acceptance that calm is good and you can remain calm confident and in control.

That the birth of a baby of health and a recovery of health with greater speed is within your ability to conceive and experience.

Recap, so now you are pregnant. You know why, You definitely know how, and you have an understanding how hypnosis for child birth works, you have experienced it. You know about your body, it makes sense now, that relaxation isn't a huge ask at all, you are aware of the influence of your hormones and know how to work your nervous system in your favour at all times. Also The Love drug oxytocin is your best friend. And so are the ways to make it....

"You are proof that love before first sight does exist." — Araceli M. Ream

CHAPTER 4

Turning Fears into Faith

"Birth takes a woman's deepest fears about herself and shows her that she is stronger than them." — Unknown.

Pregnancy is one of the most beautiful times of your whole life. Six to ten people have an overwhelming fear or phobia of child birth.[5] Here you can uncover how to overcome that.

The composition of fears within you is a direct opposition to the love you have as to the certainty that it could go right. That is where turning fears into faith is the bearing of the dichotomy of 'the turn " on your beliefs becomes the real. Like the turn of a card. From a can't to a can.

The one and only time when you can carry another human in your body when you are so close to your baby.

It's one of the most beautiful experiences of your life, even when you experience common symptoms of pregnancy. You want to fully enjoy it.

This is a place of change - this is the space of enhancement of the strength within you that brings forth the life of faith and trust within you your self and your body.

One simple faith turn is all that's required.

That the uniqueness of the birthing babies process is for you to progress through you. On the strength of your knowledge and your you - ness. Because only you know what you need and want. What is right for you. It's unearthing the layers that are preventing you tuning into that and youre building that ability now. This becomes the awareness in you that will bring forth the calm and competence that will enhance the experience for you. That enhances the experience of birth by being centered. When the fear rises we become de centred and the sense of intactness seems to shake.

You can stay intact. Just by knowing that will happen you can choose to stay intact. Emotionally, physically, increasing your sense of strength in knowledge a special approach to the education of your mind to enhance you what your body can achieve when the work in harmony. What you mind conceives your body can achieve.

These are real and may include or perpetuate the feeling of discomfort. They do not track or trail the fear and resolving the fears can begin to make them also resolve to also resolve to become strengths. That's the turn. You hear that it's a fear before you get lost in it's track. Your fear can become faith. Then turn the fear into faith, because behind a fear is a doubt and under the doubt there is a trust that is hidden because of some thing or time, so when the trust is reminded to you, you can once again regain the faith. Because it's different now.

So you can become strong and your fears can begin to resolve.

And dissolve, when the fear becomes faith then the calm becomes confidence.

Causes and sources of fear.

The known

The known of what will happen

Sometimes, the vacancy of knowledge welcomes the bliss of faith and other times it is a vacuum for fear. We set to encourage the space that makes the fears to become appropriate and maintain essential fear mechanisms whilst strengthening the sense in you that makes the fears be less dominant.

Fear is essential in many ways because it has a purpose. We are looking at the fears in context of childbirth.

The fear that something may be wrong that would spur you to take an action to contact your midwife that is appropriate. That is appropriate. But doesn't need to be experienced to the extreme. You know what is happening you know what to do and remain calm until you know.

We are talking about the deeper seated fears which compromise your ability to birth your baby with ease. These are the ones were often not aware of.

This type of fear connected in constellation that you have beliefs attached such as that you are not supported you are not loved you aren't enough... these typical beliefs on a level compound the fears and would interrupt the response of the body and mind. These would influence your intactness.

A seeming not enoughness a lacking or insufficiency of something in some way (which we all are on some levels which is part of the natural course of life to seek more) through when the instinctive drive becomes internalised to reduce the attainment of the very thing you are moving through being as you had intended then that's not helpful. And can be resolved and rewired and redirected into a more helpful thought and belief path. You are enough to birth baby. Whilst being calm, confident and in control.

So to flush through them enables a greater flow of the possible solutions. Which would in effect prove the contrary, that you are supported you are loved and there is provided before. You actual evidence that that is so.

You did have pain

The unknown that there is a lack of education or knowledge or even ignorance of what is known.

Regional sources of fears

Past experiences

Birth

Pregnancy

Labour

The potentials and so many that we can't conceivably control when you think about them – ie, the what could go wrongs (focus on the what could go rights)

That your partner isn't there

That you birth alone

That the birth plan doesn't happen as you wanted

That you won't be enough as. A mother, father

What to do when you are in labour

How to birth baby

Losses Unplanned emergency

That ..... all of the things (everyone has their own)

All of the things that you as a woman who is to birth are fearing.

Systematically taking these one by one is futile because they all stem from one pivotal point.

The words, (I heard them on an episode of Greys anatomy by Dr Bailey and other places.) and they are very very powerful when intended correctly.

> **" That** (past event) **was then, and this** (relate
> to how far you have come) **is now"**

All of these could happen. BUT you will be intact, knowing exactly what to do should they happen.

That there is a doubt within you that you are not any one of the following. They are within you. So just turn them and find as many reasons where you are that you can in different context.

That is that you are capable

You are able.

You are strong

You are sufficient you are more than enough

You are able.

> **"This is now,** (relate to how far you have come)
> **and that** (where you intend to be) **is then"**

And that you are all of the enough- ness, the enoughness to be enough and the enoughness to know that you can fill the gaps where you aren't enough because you are enough. The more you think it the more you become it.

Being enough doesn't mean doing it all, being it all, all of the time. It includes gifts dormant until required. You don't have to show up as "it all" every day and that's the magic of faith. You are there when you need to be.

It also means being enough to ask for help. And to accept help. And what you need will be there, however you allow that to happen.

To accept the help and also accept that the assistance is a symptom of your enoughness by the ability to call it forth, with grace. It's unimaginable for many the effects of Past loss trauma and past experiences. Past times when something has gone wrong. Though they are very real for some.

They offer learnings from losses of infants and the commonality within the healing of the loss is the finding of the meaning that there was a point of change in their lives and propulsion forward to make something beautiful after what would have happened.

Others, beautifully positioned … The sentiment that each child chooses its parents and it chose this particular parentage and this time and this moment to come to life and for whatever reason of life purpose they were here brought here for is helpful. Inclusive that if they choose their time to come they chose their time to leave also. They come for the learnings and experiences to the mother father and to themselves to progress the evolution and progression of the soul. When we ask why me. It's a joyful response in they chose to share their limited life with you. You were their one. Their person to bring that love to. You to be the host to their body for that time so they could experience life within you to the point they chose to leave. They didn't leave as a body because you did anything wrong they left as a body because their lessons had been learned and their lifetime as complete in this form. There is no sense in guilt or punishment. But their love and your love for them will always be within you.

They chose you to share their time on earth with you , they chose you because you were the one for them.

They chose to leave because the evolution for their soul have progressed as far as it could in this lifetime and had served its purpose it had served its purpose and was time for it to go.

But it chose you to experience on earth with and that was the bond of love that was shared between you and always will be. Somehow it takes the rawness of the emotional call when they leave. The primal yearning and the emptiness and the absolute desolation that comes with the loss of a pregnancy or baby. Again you can ask, what would you know, what about you, have you lost a baby. Yes. more than one. But I am also graced with two incredible children and the wisdom to reconcile loss in a way that brings great blessings into life. With the healing power of forgiveness.

There is always something very potent that causes the individual to change their life in some way. And if they don't, that's when the trauma sets in and the loss becomes something relived. As a message from their soul to live on once you have grieved the loss. When trauma lingers the message is being ignored.

A learning

Including miscarriage and still birth.

I do know of many women who have experienced births that would have been seen as traumatic. Having used birthing babies approaches through pregnancy and to her emotional release techniques following their losses and trauma have been resolved to have healthy successful pregnancies and great joy in them also. So the extended trauma response is avoided, even healed as they go. As they move forward it heals.

Moving forward when you remember

> " That (past event) was then, and this (relate
> to how far you have come) is now"

Fixation of attention on what there is to fear isn't helpful. So look forward and imagine something good no matter how you have lost in the past. Imagine towards the things that you haven't lost.

> "This is now, (relate to how far you have come) and
> that (where you intend to be) is then"

Because we fear what we do not know, education is key. The more you learn the less you fear.

Though everything is to be taken in balance.

I believe that the female body is designed to birth babies comfortably. To unlearn some things and relearn others

Dick Grantly reed suggests the Dick reed method

Passionately he cites " the methods are designed to protect women from the appalling dangers of ignorance"

Devised in the 1930s this method was brought to in the times when chemical intervention was the norm, archaic practices and close to butchery, when women are encourages to lay flat and sometimes basic ignorance of the anatomy of the human body and its natural functions.

The method includes breathing techniques and relaxation exactly as birthing babies does. All of the central Hypnotherapy / Alternative childbirth Methods have At least three things in common.

1. Fixation on one point.
2. Breathing techniques
3. Relaxation

These three things are common in all approaches
Because they are effective.

It's a natural consequence of life that sometimes complications happen and situations become emergent within these emergent situations there will always be one overriding factor of importance.

When you stay calm confident and in control then both you and baby have the best chances of safe passage through labour and birthing into motherhood and to meeting your baby.

So the methods here enshrined are now more pertinent and potent in their uses and can firmly be established as an asset.

They queried and questioned how many women had an episiotomy over the weeks and month. It was a high number. This is required when there is tension. If you use the image of expanding the cervix. Opening like a flower and the circular diagram then you are more able to spread the feeling of relaxation and enjoy rather than endure the feeling of being able to some extent control the physical sensations in your physical body.

No other natural bodily function is painful and childbirth should not be an exception.

When we make comparisons such as the size of a baby versus the size of an average faecal movement (I know wholly inappropriate but it is also something that have a muscular reflex pattern in the nervous system to excrete and a similar bodily system) But then, it's ok, because everybody Poos. But it's the repeated trying to imagine how something so large can exit such a small opening that makes, a basis for fear when actually in reality the capacity of the opening to stretch is immeasurable.

In sphincter responses: Stress effects both- Tension effects both - Both are effected

When you can't wee in places when theres people listening it is not the physical function it's the fear and judgment around it so when this is no longer the focus of attention, you are distracted or you are attentive to the actual process of weeing rather than the source of the fear, as a matter of importance you can wee. Example - A woman was in an outside toilet at a pub, and could only hear the jovial chatter and it felt like the people were listening. Nervous bladder, you know this. She asked her boyfriend to sing, refusing to come out until he did, sing outside the door so she could pee. It works. You are asking your mind to stop worrying about who is listening and to just wee, with distraction with a different fixation. Ultimately you are choosing where your attention goes with grows with the intactness and the hue. And then comes the calm balance. The fixation of your attention is moulded by hypnotherapy for childbirth. Inwardly it's more comfortable.

Other bodily functions where pain is induced by stress or fear. The fear of the pain itself causes the tension and makes it worse. The fear of the pain is often the source of the tension and actually with controlled movement there is improvement.

I remember a time when I was walking. I slipped on a coast path to a hidden beauty spot, it was stunning , but as a landed I felt movement in my ankle. Like a click. I carried on, even though I knew something wasn't ok. I carried on calmly It felt like walking on a stump in retrospect.

(As luck would have it I was in the days preceding recording the audio sequences so had been reciting pain control Hypnotherapy paradigms) So it is no wonder I activated spontaneously the sensation of comfort to get me home to safety. And to make a point there was no danger in this affect. I walked home about two miles with company, when I returned to the car and sat I suddenly I felt the sensation something was wrong, I drove home and tried to walk on my foot and realised it had swollen to three to four times it is natural size in the time I had been travelling in the car. I went for an x - ray - Just a sprain, crutches, predicted 6 weeks on crutches. I made this down to three days with meditation and directed intention. And you can too. Expediate the healing. The audios work.

The Science of fear

Cortisol increases. Sympathetic nervous arousal where tension exists in the body and it's less easy to make for the body to flow and circulate around the system

The aim

To be calm, confident and in control

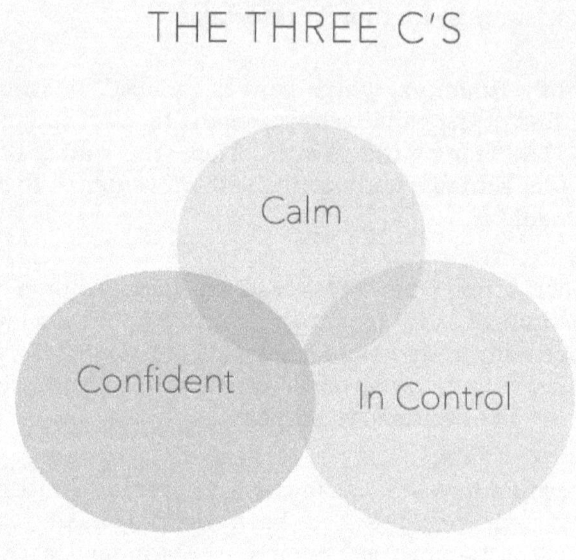

Assuming the antidote to fear is love. The essential allies in overcoming the pattern of love inhibiting fears.

The Physical ways

Breathing

The reasons why, include more Oxygenated blood increases the efficiency of muscles in labour also efficiency of muscles and organs in pregnancy. Circulating more oxygenated blood around the body is much more effective.

Lymphatic drainage and promotes the release of waste products from body. The Flow of oxygenated blood into the uterine muscles and direct to baby filling every cell with vital oxygen.

Feels better, Gives you More energy, Cleansing for you body and you feel fresher more alert, Before during and after labour, Activates lymphatic drainage stimulates the lymph system, Activates weight loss post pregnancy – by activating the internal metabolism.

Brings a greater sense of good health and balance out the emotional resonance of your body. You can use one of two methods.

Box breathing

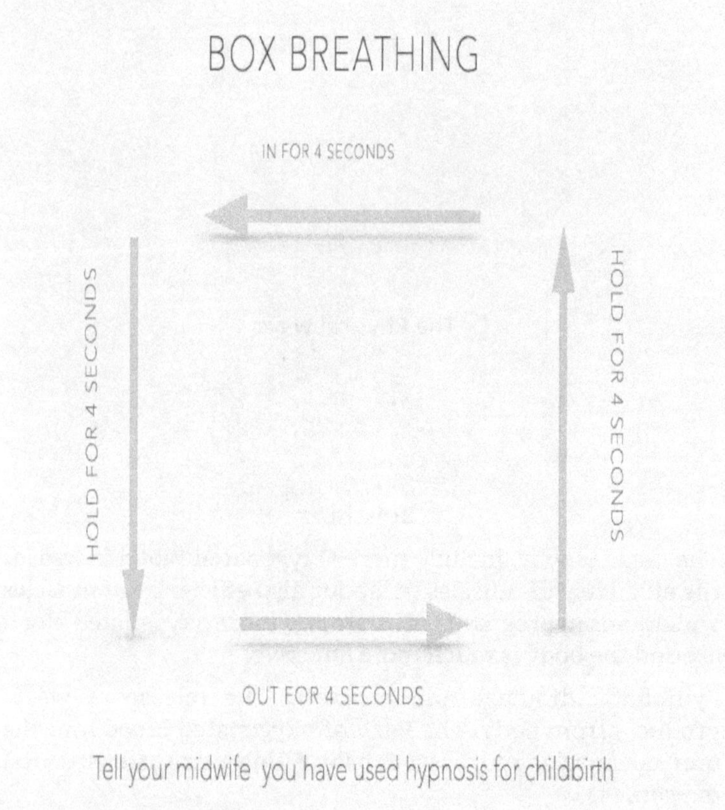

Calming rhythm of breath with four points of focus. In ....
two three four ....hold.... two three four ....Out ...two three
four....Hold...Two Three four

Diaphramatic breathing where you tense your throat muscles as you breathe out to make a " ahh " sound. At the back of your throat.

This breath has a ratio of 1: 2

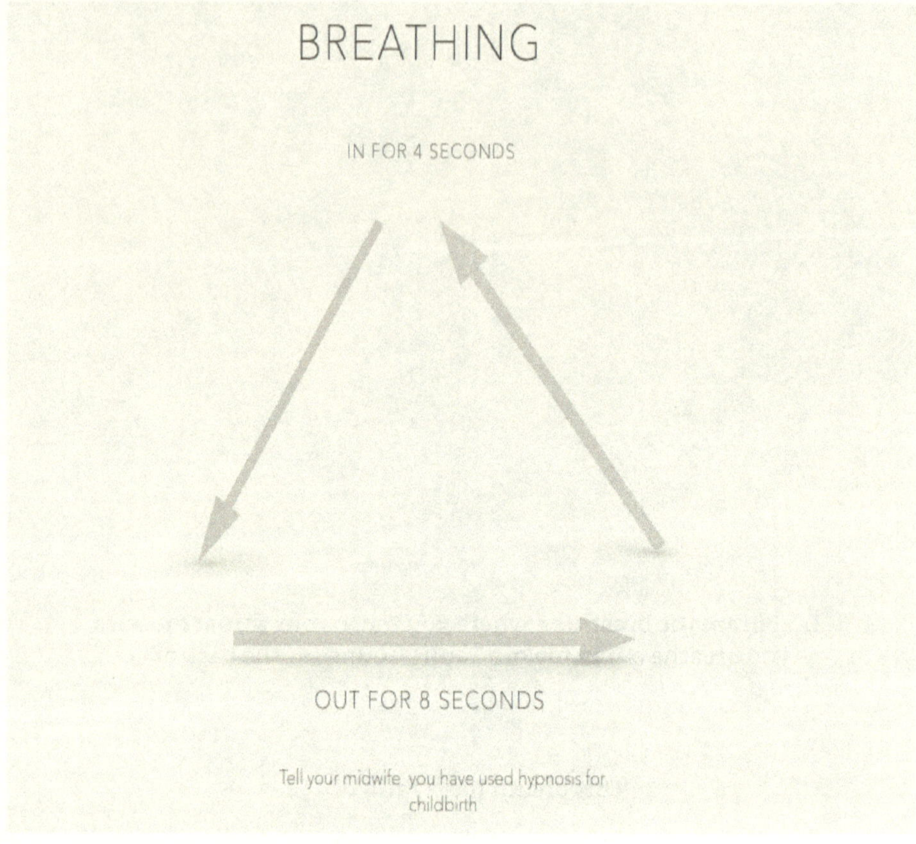

**All in breathing techniques with enable you to centred.
Oxygenate your body and bring you health.**

The Mental ways

Awareness of the fear tension pain cycle - Calm ease flow - Fixation of attention

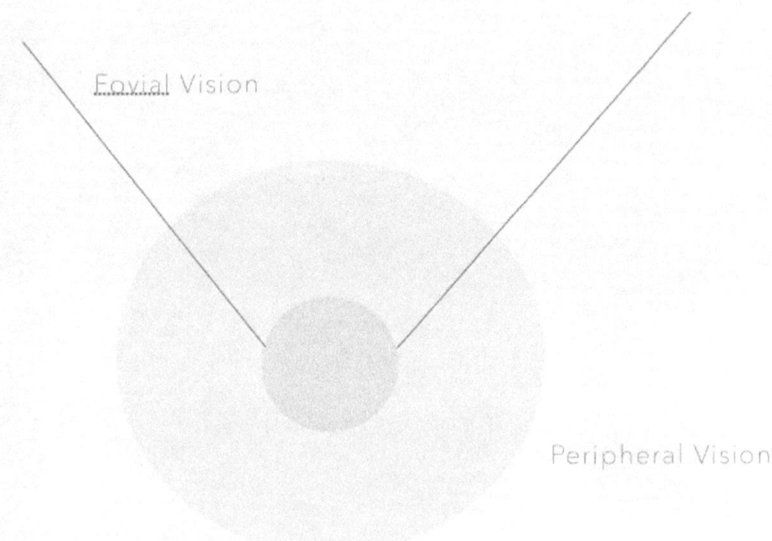

Using peripheral vision allows us to process pre consciously. We are unconsciously aware of our environment inspecting and converging billions of sensory perceptions to form the perceive your experience of the living world.

When you are already aware of so much more of your surroundings you have less concept of the fears because within the sensory experience of the space you are in it does not escalate a far as the sensory review from your resonation with the environment evaluated that there is no situation to fear in clouding the consideration of what is occurring within your body not just for external perceptions.

Fixation on a central point above the eyes and becoming aware of the space around you the room around you. Focus on a spot on the wall and fixate upon it. As if you can imagine a ball at the back of your head and are able to sense 360 degrees while still fixating on the spot. You will feel a sense of calm a sense of relief. That's good. Then bring your eyes down into the room you are in and move forward with your day without questioning the feeling.

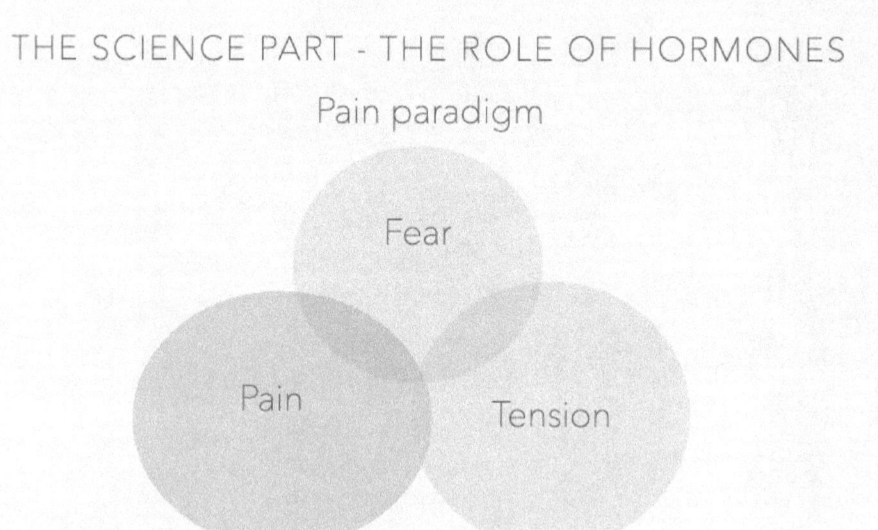

The Emotional Ways

When we think of strength it's easy to imagine masculine form. And to be women ourselves have the sense in the finite beauty that is a woman and that is ok. Femininity does not mean weakness, in fact it symbolises great strength.

But it's also to embody the presence of the strength of a woman with the finesse and composure. Child birth can resemble this and embody this. It calls forward something in you that is beyond rational thought. Because it is a primal function. The unseen unknown strength you have. It's primal and instinctive. But it is also calm and composed.

In two ways. The fears begin to move and become strengths great strengths when they have the right movement and turn around them.

But in some ways you can rise around them. Move through them and what makes that possible is the strength of your will and faith in your body and faith in your mind.

Both routes provide strength and comfort in their form in movement in the acceleration of progression as you trust in your body and the fears subside or even dissolve.

The fears you have are founded somewhere Somewhere within you and for the fear to exist so much the comparison as there was once a time when the fear didn't exist. So it's not to find the fear backwards but knowing what you know now would the fear still exist. Probably not. So as you move through the book. Those fears can dissolve and become learnings and understandings. And that can establish a sense of permanence within you.

You will feel your thoughts turn. Things will make sense as to the questions that you hadn't dared to ask being answered by the revelation of the information you see before you when it resonates within your mind it becomes a new valued truth not to before held but to find resolution and comfort within.

Within you and there is a specific induction within the birthing babies audio series specifically designed to combat these. Sources below [6][7]

They are an essential aspect of your preparation for birth.

Acceptance of your mind being more malleable by affirmation of self belief becoming stronger more centered and more coherent as a woman who births with strength grace and confidence.

Similarly when

Your fears are founded in you by something of a past memory or a symptom of the influence of your environment upon you. They are overcome able and discernible, and they are changeable.

Fears present a systematic process that is all. They pervade calm. They elude calm. Calm and fear cannot co exist so when the fear is of the known – what has happened in the past then the antidote to the resolution of the fear is appreciating the difference between the then and the now. Two times. Two spaces. Two places. And it's different now.

Also knowing what you know now would you have even felt the fear in the first place. Maybe not. Once again.

Evaluation of the separation by time, knowledge, learning and personal growth.

When you imagine a time in the future when the event fear has been for told and happened with its completion at the resolution that you had hoped for instead of feared then the balance of the faith begins to move.

You observe what you hope for with greater intent and determination. Each time you observe the fear. Remembering they are your fears and therefore it is your mind they stem from and therefore it is you who can change them. Redirect them reassure them that they aren't required and intend the observation of the event as you would determine it to you. Listening to the audios will also help.

So, the turn on your perspective.

Just by using the intentions time and time again –

Turn fears into confidences... it will happen. Repeat the sentence within.

Turn insecurity into security

Turn fear into faith

Turn anxiety into excitement and hope

Turn overload into calm confidence

Turn doubt into certainty

Turn lack into plenty

Turn weak into strength

Turn hurt into loved

Turn rejected into accepted

Turn unsupported into supported

Turn lost into healed, intact.

Turn ..... into ....

The more you intend on this exercise the more potent it becomes

Mentally take a breath and relax.

Then close your eyes and repeat the list to yourself.

Turn ..... into ......

Also the future envisioning

Imagine 20 minutes after the event you fear and retrospectively glance towards now with a sense that everything has gone well then return your perspective to now and back to the point beyond the thing you were anxious about and then think about and notice how it feels different.

Repeat – try this with something innocuous in your everyday life and notice how it works very effectively.

For example parking spaces.

Imagine worrying about parking – 20 minutes after getting to your destination imagining how easy it was to find parking then

Imagine getting to your destination from now

The way you anticipate will change and the route you take may change

You may imagine a new space to park or a different solution and a solution will present itself to you the more you use this envisioning technique.

Then the intentions are relaid and relay new pathway of certainty and faith. The through time become you and that is so.

And keep going.

The space in between these will correct itself as you intend it more.

But it starts with the intention to turn. To Change.

Because you intend more because you intend.

Without the intention to turn the fear that is to become faith there is no movement in the space of the fear it remains static and very much there. Niggling.

When you are in the space of relaxation and the fixation of attention, your attention is fixated on the calm confidence. The niggles go.

When you are in the appreciation of the strength of your body as a miracle, when you are in appreciation of the reflex, which presents the beginning of your labour, already ordained within you it is already within you to birth. The more you marvel at the miracle of you with whilst retaining the pragmatism of everyday life you can appreciate your ability to overcome fear. And the fear turns into strength. It literally turns. The perspective changes. The frame of reference changes and becomes different when you change your perspective the experience of the fear changes. And becomes more a centered composure. Because it is different. It becomes a strength. core strength. That is how the faith turn effects.

So begin

List the things you fear

List the things they represent lacking in you and then list what you see is missing in you.

If you can perceive it there is a chance it already exists within you

Pain imagine turning it into comfort

Anxious turn it into calm

Fear - turn it into a sense of competence calm

Uncertainty tun into calm competence preparedness

You can also do a scaled approach

Where the turn is too great you can use a polarity scale

You can do the same with the dials

Imagine a series of dials in an internal control panel for confidence turn up the dial for confidence.

Turn the dial for satisfaction after a meal – so you don't overeat to discomfort

Turn down the dial of discomfort in your body

Imagine dials for security – turn up the dials and see new possibilities become apparent for you

Each and every one will open up more possibility.

Imagine dials

For pain sensation (as is spoken in the audios)

Anything that has a polarity can have a dial.

Everything that has a spectrum can have a dial.

Imagine 15 minutes after giving birth holding baby and know that you are ok baby is ok and know you have done and that you are more than you ever thought you could possibly be.

"You are proof that love before first sight does exist." — Araceli M. Ream

ALLOW YOUR EYES TO GENTLY CLOSE

Just let the outside world simply fade away

Give your thoughts time to become still and quiet

Notice whatever sound you can hear around you

Maybe the sounds of the music in the back ground

Maybe the gently ticking of a clock

Maybe even the sound of the air moving within the room

Be aware of the sound of your own breathing

Allow these sounds to become part

Of your experience

Allow them to become more important to you

Imagine that there is a little person inside your mind

And that little person is sweeping up all of the worries the cares

The words

The thoughts and the concerns of the day

Gently blow the dust away in the quietness and the stillness
that is left imagine that you are at the beginning of your
labour its now time for your baby to be born

Nothing is expected of you

There is nothing you have to do

You don't even have to listen to my voice

You don't need to do anything but to enjoy the feelings that come

To enjoy the feelings of relaxation that increase with every breath you take

And increasing with each word that I speak

Gently focus into your breathing

Notice the gentle rise and fall of your chest

With each easy breath

Imagining breathing the calmness

And breathing out the tension

Breathing in calmness

And breathing out tension

Just like a sigh

If calmness had a colour

Imagine what that colour would be for you

What would the colour of calm be for you
If contentment had a colour what colour would that be for you.

See it

Sense it

Feel it

Imagine yourself surrounded by that colour of calm just
like a warm swirling soothing mist of calm each tie you
breathe in you are breathing in that colour of calm

If tension had a colour

Imagine what that colour would be

What would the colour of tension be for you

See it sense it

Feel it

Imagine breathing out that t colour of tension

As you are breathing in that colour of calmness

Breathing out the colour of tension

Breathing in calmness

And breathing out tension

Just like a sigh

Find your own natural rhythm feel those breaths
in reaching right down to your baby

Soothing your baby

Sending positive messages to your baby

That everything is well

Acting like a very soothing anesthetic

Breathing yourself down into peacefulness

Down into calm ness

Down into stillness of mind

Experience your body reacting to this deep relaxation

Imagine that you are standing in a beautiful path of rain forest

This lush rainforest runs along by a beautiful stretch of sandy beach

You have been walking through the resin forest in the direction of the each

The last bit of inclined forest path

This lush rain forest runs along a beautiful stretch of sandy
beach you have been walking through the rain forest in the
direction of the beach the last bit of inclined forest path will
eventually lead you out into the sandy shores of the beach

But before you leave the rain forest you stop and stand

And look above and take in the lush greens and take in the canopy of the lush
rain forest trees you can see the strong sunlight beaming through the foliage

Like rays of glistening energy

You can hear exotic birds

And sounds that soothe you with a reminder that
nature s happening all around

The smell of the air is crisp clean and fresh and
alive with wonderful exotic smells

The birds are singing so happily and chattering to other birds in the forest

You take-in a few deep breaths to smell the abundant rain forest aromas

Anda as you breathe out

Relax - deeper and deeper

And as you continue on your way

Yo come to a winding pathway whch leads you out of a

Down onto the beach

It may be one which is familiar to you

Or one which you have constructed in your imagination

Notice how eager you are to descent to the beach

The sand

Looks golden and inviting

And as you descend

I will count from ten down to one

And you will be standing on the beach

Start descending down onto the beach

Ten

Nine

You are getting closer to your beach

Eight

Seven

You are feeling more

Six

Five

More an more relaxed

Four almost there

Three

Two

You are now standing on the beach feeling very relaxed and happy

The beach is everything you dreamed it to be

Stretching out before you is miles of incredible white golden sand

As you slowly walk along relaxing deeper and deeper with each step

Notice what you are wearing

You are feeling confident

And comfortable

As you slip of your shoes stretch and stroll across the gold
sand you feel the warm sand under the soles of your feet
you can see the grains glistening in the sunlight

There is no one but you here

Simply enjoying some precious time to yourself

You stand and gaze at the incredible view

The brilliant mixes of jade green and iridescent views of the ocean foreshore

You gaze out into the distance of the calm blue sea

And see the vastness stretching out before you

Marveling at the spaciousness and the sense of freedom

There is a fishing boat in the distance with its colorful sail

Gently bobbing up and down

The sun is shining

The sky is blue

And not a cloud in sight

Take a moment to notice what gentle sound you can hear

Perhaps there are some seagulls in the distance

Perhaps you can hear the peaceful a lapping of the waves

Perhaps you can hear your own gentle breathing

Perhaps you can hear your own

Take a few moments to notice hat else you an hear

You are embarking on one of the most incredible experiences of your life

you are feeling so relaxed and you r howl body feels
comfortably loose and limp and relaxed

You hear the sounds of your leaves and your whole body feels relaxed

The breeze keeps your face cool and the sun
continues to energies your whole body

And you watch how the waves roll towards the beach

In a never ending sequence one after another and then
petering y=out as they near the beach

You walk towards the waters edge

Witnessing the immense power of nature enabling the waves
to move forward before receding into the wet sand

And when you reach the sea you gently let your toes test the water

Which is slightly cool as you take few more steps into the
water you are feeling the immense power of nature

A normal natural process

And as you allow the waves to roll over your feet and ankles and retreat again

You breathe in the salty sea air and relax deeper and deeper

As you allow the waves to roll over you r feet and
ankles and then retreat again

You breathe in the fresh salty sea air

And relax deeper.

You realize that just like the surging of the waves is a process you can see
and feel so what is happening in your body is a normal natural process

A physiological process that your body knows how to do

You walk as far as the small waves

Where you let your feet feel the cool washes of the
water the water washes over your ankles

They roll in like delicate rushes of energy

As the waves within your own body become more powerful

It is a constant reminder that you an trust your body

I trust my body it knows what to do

You feel a growing feeling of peace and calm

As the warm sea air lightly brushes your skin

And as your feet sink into the sand beneath the
water with every step you take

So you are relaxing deeper and deeper with each step

And you notice much the sea is up close

As wave after wave rolls up towards you

Each contraction will bring me closer towards the birth of my baby

Each contraction has its own job to do

Once that contraction has gone I will never be able
to experience that contraction again

Each contraction in your body

Each one a reminder that your body knows what to do

I trust my body it knows what to do

Labour is a normal

Physiological process

The natural moments of the waves remind you of the
a natural movements within your body

As you notice a contraction within your body

You tilt your head slightly upwards towards the sun

You feel the suns energy and light all over your face

It feels like the sun its there for you and for no one else

The feeling brings a small smile to your face

And you instinctively know all is well within your body and with your baby

Nothing in the world is bothering you now

Any small worries or anxieties leave your mind as they surface –

Watch them drift out to sea

On the gentle breeze after a while you stroll back up the beach to
a most inviting deck chair which sit there especially for you

And there is a sunshade and a table

And your favorite refreshing drink

And as you adjust the sunshade so it is just right for you

As you lies back in the chair and you relax deeper
and deeper still and you breathe out

When you need hydration your body send clear messages
to drink water to refresh and revitalize you

When you need something more for your baby your body will send
a clear and comfortable sign to look towards a professional

While sitting there identify any worries you have at this time about labour
about child birth and parent hood imagine them leaving your mind and
coming back as learnings , integrations or solutions and new options

As they float away on the wind out to sea telling yourself the
worries have now gone as you lie there on the warm sand
with the sea breezes washing over your face you notice your
breathing has slowed down to a comfortable pace

Your breathes are less frequent

Your whole body is safe warm and

Your mind is calm

Youre at peace

I trust my body

It knows what to do

And because you are so calm our body will be free to progress
your labour and your baby will be calm also

For now enjoy the sea breezes and enjoy the warmth of the sun

Spend as long as you want on your beach before taking three deep breaths
and exhaling fully before starting to breathe at your usual rate again

Wriggle your fingers and your toes

This will help your mind to renter your body

And when you fee ready

Slowly open your eyes

And take a few moments to enjoy the calm and relaxed
feelings that now linger over you

And notice your environment and the people around you

Retaining tat sense of calm and knowing that you can return to your
beach by counting down from ten to one whenever it feels right to do so

This incredible experience is just short way into the future
leaving you some time to visit your beach

Building up anticipation and excitement about this time with your baby

But for now

I am going to count

From one

To ten

And as I do you will feel more and more alert

More and more refreshed

Confident in the knowledge that you can do this

A renewed faith in yourself and your body

One

Two

C SECTIN REHEARSAL SCRIPT
Relaxation session 3

(COPYRIGHT - VICTORIA WHITNEY –
BIRTHING BABIES © 2023)

Simply close your eyes and let everything else fade away in importance

I want you to think of the word relax ……

Think about how it has two syllables

Re lax…

As you breathe in think

Re to yourself

And as you breathe out

Think lax

Don't let your mind wander away for repeating the word relax

When you breathe out try to let go of any tension in your body

Focus on those muscles, which may have been holding some tension

Every time you breathe out lax the out breath is the one to focus on

The in breath takes care of itself

Think re on each breath in and lax on each breath out

Imagine those out breaths

Are being blown into a big balloon all of your tensions

being expelled from your body and being blown into that big balloon

The balloon being filled up with air and when it is full imagine it floating away

And as it floats away the balloon carries away all of those tensions

And you Reeel aaaax You reee laaaax

Calm confident and in control

Each breath

And you are feeling completely in control

Allow your hands to rest comfortably on top of your legs wherever they feel most comfortable

Now as you relax more and let it go ore and more

You can allow every muscle in your body to relax

Every cell every nerve every fiber in your body relaxing

Now picture in your mind a candle this candle can be any color you with it to be

The color you have chose n for your candle is a color you unconscious mind knows relaxes you and calms your mind

Calms you and relaxes your mind. It is your color of calm

Now focus on you the color of the flame of the candle

See how amazing the colors within the flame are

You may see red, blue yellow purple white

And maybe another color

And as you see the colors within the flame you relax more and more

And go deeper

And as you enjoy these heavy and relaxed feelings deeply relaxed feelings

These feelings of being in control.

Now focus on the wax body of your candle

Now see the first trickle of melting wax begin to move down the wax

Now see the melting wax touch the candleholder and merge with it to become part of the candleholder

You become more and more relaxed

Feeling safe and comfortable

Now imagine that you re that candle

A candle of total relaxation

Now within this relaxation you can think towards a safe place inside

Within that safe place you will have a space to build ne experience of the unknown.

You can imagine now that you are within the preparation for your theatre you are prepared and feeling calm confident and in control your re surrounded by professionals who know what to do to help you birth your baby

So you can be calm confident and in control

The room smells clinical and that's of comfort, as you know it's a safe way to right baby on this day

The sounds the colors you can acclimatize very quickly

You remember the candle the candle of ultimate relaxation

Any nerves or fears can simply dissolve as you have a sense of comfort and priority to bright baby with ease faith love ad safely maintaining that sense of comfort always knowing that you are doing the right thing for you and the right thing for abbey

And you remember the candle the candle of ultimate

relaxation and feel calm confident and in control

The sense of the room is professional and clean though you have the sense of growing warmth and love within you building and building and feeling of greater comfort

You move towards the theater and as you go rethought doors you can small the clean and fresh environment you can sense the setting is ok, it is safe and you feel comfortable to proceed with the procedure

As you prepare you may be required to lie down or sit upon the edge of the bed for a small numbing treatment. It feels totally normal. It feels totally comfortable. You know what to expect. You are calm confident and in control any fears or worries can just release as you breathe in calm and breathe out tension breathe in calm and breathe out tension

As you do you feel calm confident and strong within

Each moment is taking you closer to birthing your baby safely

Each and every breath you take is bringing you closer to birthing your baby so you enter into the theatre and you lie on the table

The clothes and gowns and masks feel appropriate and you have a growing sense of comfort knowing that each moment is bringing you closer to birthing your baby

You can hear the instruments whirring in the background and the light are bright and that feels comfortable

You have a sense of warmth and comfort within you through you and around you and a strong sense also to enjoy the experience of birthing baby

To be aware and to be alive and to feel the comfortable sense of calm confident awareness growing within you

As you look up and see the gowns and the doctors at their work you may hear the tinkling of the medical instruments in the room and each moment and each sound that you recognize gives you a deepening sense of comfort and sense of control within that comfort knowing that each breath and each moment that passes is bringing you closer to birthing your baby as time passes the surgeons may speak with you and update you they will guide you so you know what is happening moment by moment

And the sense of comfort within you remains strong with each breath in.

As you take one now and relax knowing that everything is ok

And you remember the candle the candle of ultimate relaxation and feel calm confident and in control

As you hear the sound of the tinkling instruments and you may feel sense of pressure under your ribs just before baby is born

As you do you breathe in and relax and allow the process to continue knowing that each moment and each breath brings you closer to birthing your baby

Any discomfort you can remember the candle within and the dials the internal dials to switch down the discomfort once it's message has been heard you can turn the dials down

Then you can hear the sound of your baby's cry as you imagine looking up and baby is there. So your body can now begin to synthesize the hormone oxytocin the love drug because it can and it can increase the sense of love and healing for your body and for bonding with baby. The moment you hear baby's cry's and see baby your body responds to the birth with the production of the love hormone so you can accelerate your physical healing and from bond with baby and move through the coming hours days and weeks with a strong sense of love bonding with baby, feeding baby, and the sense of closeness and completion.

And you remember the candle, the candle of ultimate relaxation and feel calm confident and in control as you see the candle in your minds eye you know your body is healing and using it energy and nutrients to birth you and baby

Your body can heal and is healing every breath you now take without conscious thought or effort you are now healing renewing

Bond with a baby and feel baby on your skin your body's natural response immediately as baby bonds with you bond with baby and feel that deepening sense of strength and comfort as you progress the sense of comfort you have is deepening and beginning fill your whole body that sense of great love and joy combined as the relief that baby is here

There resting on your chest

You can smell them and feel their tiny arms and legs moving now outside of your body and the beauty of the experience is all encompassing

The love with you and baby and that moment will be within you for the whole of your life together and always be safe and protected in your mind and remembered when needed so you can stay calm confident and in control if you ever experience a sense of unease or not enough ness you can remember that bond that strength that love and that love will move you forward to make the very best things happen .

And you take a deep breath in and this memory begins to fade but it fades into moments and seconds of your future time and living memory so it becomes to the future so you can stay firmly present in the now and enjoy each moment of life throughout.

And as you do you can remaining very relaxed take a few moments to breathe in and out and in

And out and then as I count form one to 10 on the number ten you will awaken alert and in the room.

One

Two

Three

Four

Five

Six

Seven

Eight

Nine

Ten

Recap, so now you are pregnant. You know why, You definitely know how, and you have an understanding how hypnosis for child birth works, you have experienced it. You know about your body, it makes sense now, that relaxation isn't a huge ask at all, youre aware of the influence of your hormones and know how to work your nervous system in your favour at all times. Also The Love drug oxytocin, it is your best friend. And so are the ways to make it.... You know the science of fear, how to reduce it, You have the mental ways the physical ways and the environmental ways. You knowhow to influence your hormone balance and reduce stress hormones to the positive for the purpose you have for birthing babies. You know how to breathe, you know how to You have overcome many fears, and turned them into confidences. You know how to breathe, forever to bring you calm. You have a confidence prelude to a c sections even if it is unplanned.

CHAPTER 5

LABOUR

"Giving birth is an incredible act of nature and power." - Michele Obama.

I t's show time .....

Traditionally the phases of labour are broken down into stages. As your progress can be measured and you will know where you are in relation to your babies birth.

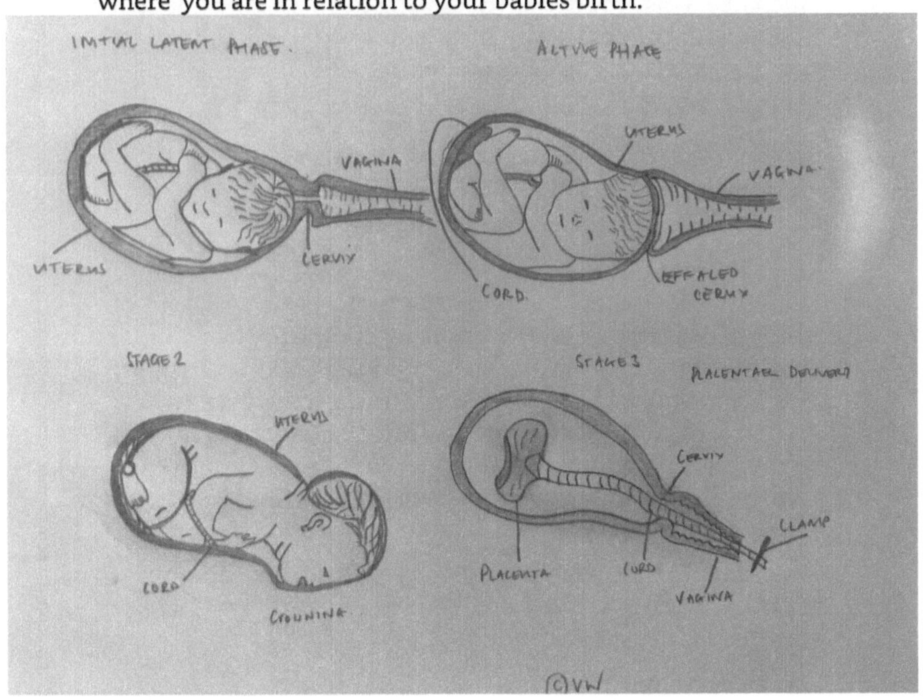

STAGE ONE

First stage of labour

Common experiences will include....

Body heat will rise or drop

You will urge to empty bladder

Hiccup or feel nauseated as your body begins to shift around the activity in your uterine muscles.

These aren't exclusive and there are many many more.

You will have the sense for the need to escape, possibly as a reverse flow of the babies sensations to you. How sometimes people suggest that you have personality changes when you are in pregnancy like you have waves of the soul of the baby.

The waves of the personality of the baby.

Much like when your body moves you towards the same space in you will feel that sense of urgency to escape though you could interpret this as baby is coming.

And a desire to find a safe space to begin the process of labouring baby.

Your sense of time will become distorted you will be so focussed and absorbed. Into the process.

Like ultra marathon runners. The best ones I know do not check their watches. Do not check with time because they are so at one with the run that they just keep going it is as if it is another world, to them they are running. Like when you are working. You are on task. No rest stop. Therefore the run has a life of it is own. From start to finish they are running and the only thing that is of matter to them at that time is their run and being centred within the run.

Not thinking how long is left or even putting one foot in front of the other they are just one whole running. They just keep going until they get to the end.

You are birthing.

Consider this a birthing day. It's a birth day the babies first birthday that you are completely absorbed in. Your first birth day to baby. The one on all of which are built here after and you stay calm confident and in control;

Therefore you are birthing and that is what you are doing.

Time is for the midwives to monitor you are to birth, and enjoy the breathing and centering and contraction and breathing of baby down and then in turn the final moments of pushing. Is what you are doing It is as if it is one of those times in your life when you will feel completely taken care of – it is as if as you move though the book and listen to the audios your mind is going ahead and making it so.

That you are totally taken care of in all ways so that all you can do is stay centred and move forward within your life.

Transition phase - shift to birthing breathing.

Breathing down.

You are breathing down into your abdomen. You are breathing down the act of your breath and muscles working in this way will use your energy to push baby down. Pushing the uterine muscles will further the progression of labour by utilising the muscular movement to engage the muscles in the abdomen it will also calm the impulses and bring order to the chaos of the movement of the stimulus which has began the progression of labour. It gives the energy and impulses direction so you experience less of the random sensations. You are directing your attention and energy with Each breath And the progression of labour will continue with your control of your breathing in a calm confident sensation will become you.

Abdominal breathing

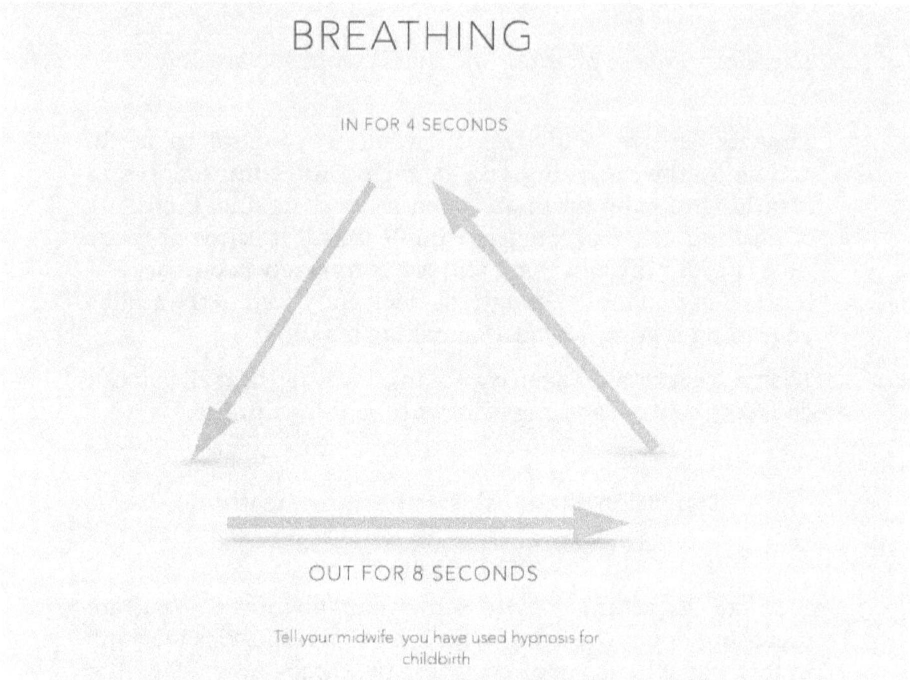

BREATHING

Deep breath in and a one to two ratio on the out breath -
the outbreath twice as long as the in breath
You can also include what is now become fashionable - box breathing

BOX BREATHING

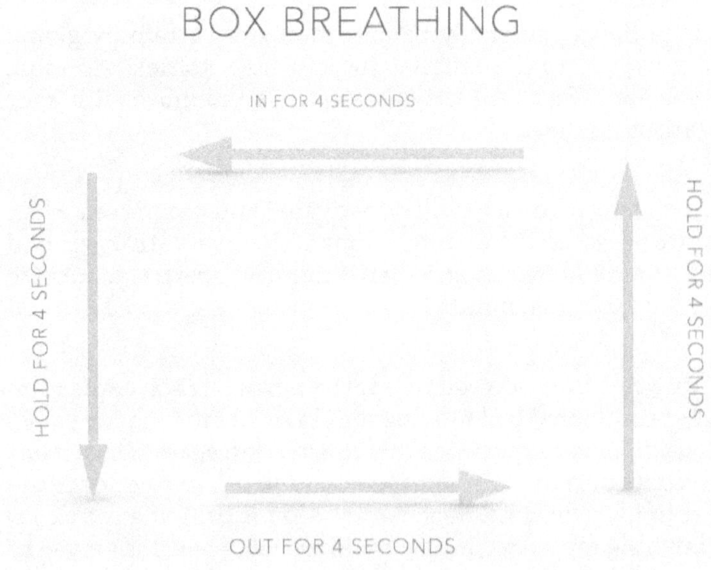

Tell your midwife you have used hypnosis for childbirth

PUSHING

At this point you are Not pushing – You are breathing the baby out.

The waves in the uterus are peristaltic waves – They are waves of movement with purpose like pulses. Any forced pushing hinders progress.

When your body wants to push the energy of the push is very powerful and comes close to the end of labour. If you have ever felt the need to push and been asked to stop pushing when your body wants to push you will understand though with these techniques you can refine and control the energy of the body inclination to push by harnessing your focus into a breath this brings your attention and central nervous system to distribute the energy by giving it another purpose. With an overwhelming physical urge to push you can this will begin to and the energy of the movement of the push to focus on your breathing to maintain the energy of movement at your control in the breath it will feel more comfortable. Very simply it gives it somewhere to go that is helpful and focussed and supports your body in birthing baby. With minimal distress.

This protects your body from unnecessary strain by giving more oxygen to the muscles in your body to flex and more as you are calm so are they as you trust and move with your breath so do they.

And the urges to push will be activated and progressed when the are necessary. The contractions at their very strongest will be 1 minute in length and then 3 minutes apart. One minute intensity to three minutes rest.

During this time you can repeat the phrase. " Each contaction is like a bouncing ball moving me closer to birthing my baby " " You will never experience this contraction again " Once it has served its purpose it is complete. And you can experience the next in it's own time. Each contraction is bringing me closer to birthing my baby. Imagine the bouncing ball. It's very very powerful.

Using breathing to control pushing. Oxygenates the muscles most importantly the perineum and will allow the perineum to be flexible because of the state of calm that pervades you.

Pushing in the later stages of delivery being calmed causes less pressure on the perineum.

This means there is a reduced risk to tear because you are working with your body. And the relaxation of your muscles and focus on the dilation of the cervix and vaginal muscles will also reduce the pressure and requirement for episiotomy.

To slow down pushing even when your body wants to and the contractions are very very strong, you can pant and breathe very very slowly exhaling as if you would only cause a candle to flicker if you were blowing into it. **Controlled breathing.**

So very gently, so very very gently.

Breathe out the excess energy of push and breath in the energy of calm breathe out the energy of push and breathe in the energy of flow breathe forward the energy of flow and gently push so the energy exertion is distributed through the control of the breath and your muscular pushing so as to reduce pressure on the vaginal walls and perineum.

Here are three intentions - you can make an image of the word push and flow and calm. Give them a colour to make this very simple.

1. Breathe out any excess, breathe out the colour of "push" and breath in the colour of calm

2.Breathe out the colour of push and breathe in the colour of flow.

3. Breathe forward the colour of flow and gently push with a candle flicker breath. A breath so light that if you were blowing onto a candle it would stay alive.

Women giving birthing in a coma with no conscious pushing at all. There are huge ecology issues maintaining pregnancy when women are in a coma or even had the experience of brain death and are on life support the principle of the point in question is that it is possible that a woman's body can birth a baby when in a coma. Though that is not to say, or imagine, it is right, Whatever the ecology issues the point in concern is that it is Possible. And huge ecology issues with a medical perspective in this. Though the principle in point it the body can do it without a conscious mind. Without the conscious control of the " host " of the body being present.

The body can birth a baby into the environment without a controlling mind. [i]

So the interception of the thoughts that would interfere with the birth being calm natural and your body birthing baby with ease is achieved as you work through this book and especially "Powerful positivity for child birth. " If we elude the thoughts that would prelude an uncomfortable birth. By way of hypnosis and relaxation with guided suggestion to the contrary then a comfortable birth should prevail. So actively focusing your consciousness on supportive mechanisms and visualisations will clear the way for a more comfortable birth.

Visualising creating sensations of calm and visualising the sensations of opening of the cervix in colour in your minds eye...are just two examples of how your mind can focus to actively support you birthing baby.

The circles each relaxing, concentric circles. Opening up like a flower with each breath of relaxation you experience. To red to orange to yellow to green and to blue. Expanding at your bodies chosen pace. As you centre your attention on the wave of each contraction concentric circles opening at your bodies chosen pace.

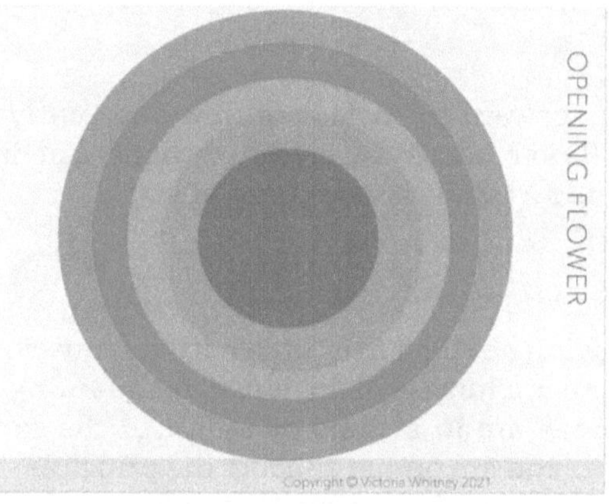

If you choose you can colour the circles by hand in this book. Own them and embed the words above.

The episiotomy is not essential nor the pushing or size of the baby nor any singular cause for the need. It is possible that the simple handling of the final stages by controlling your breath, push and body. Like reversing a really large car into a small space – add in a multistorey car park so your perception is enclosed and you have the idea. It's a precision, you can adhere and achieve through the control of your body and breathing through relaxation fixation and positioning alone. But it takes practice.

BABYS EXPERIENCE OF BIRTH

Baby starts labour by producing hormones that start the production of oxytocin.

Baby wants to breathe that is reportedly what starts the process of labour.

ORIGINAL MAGICAL MYSTERY TOUR
The pressure builds around babies head (like putting a turtle neck sweater on.) Simultaneously the pressure is also building around the babies buttocks as the uterus contracts upon them and pushes baby along through the birth canal (very sensory like being hugged from all directions) Like a massage the muscles are massaging baby through the birth canal and as they do stimulating its innate systems of independent life support to life. Waking up, the heart lungs and massaging the skin for circulation walking baby into a independent life support where its body is able to thrive outside of the womb. The massaging stimulated the babies nervous system to excrete hormones and the chemical response required to thrive outside of the womb and this all happens while baby is moving through the birth canal into this world.

Massaging the skin and encouraging the cells to bring more energy to the surface of the body.

As you consider the baby has to the time been within its amniotic sac with very little contact and stimulation from outside of its body. It will now begin to wake up within the body to having an exterior. The sensation of closeness and contact being there. Being a comfort and being a now new continuum also.

The birth canal is 23cms long

As the babies crown reaches the pelvic floor muscles they are soft and springy and are eased over the head little by little massaging.

Head up and down against firm resistance baby crowns it head, Right angled bend babies head turns and its shoulders exit the birth canal into life.

Medication

Medication is a point of contention for some. Though the purpose of Hypnotherapy for Child birth is never to evade the use of medication but to give woman choice. And ways she can find alternative should she choose. The truth and some facts about medication which will either allay any concerns you may have or cause you to choose with an educated mind. The placenta is very effective at reducing the amount of the chemicals in your body crossing into baby. Even some forms of chemotherapy are possible without harm to baby in pregnancy because they have been engineered so. Though here are some basic facts.

The central (though not exclusive) list of pain medications available in labour include.

Paracetamol- no known effects to baby

Cocodamol - no known effects to baby

Tens machines

Deliver electrical impulses to stimulate your bodies natural pain killers.

Gas and air

Oxygen and nitrous oxide gas.

Entanox – has no known negative effects for the baby

Pethidine injections

Side effects may make you feel woozy and it is an opiod there fore has addictive qualities.

Takes 20 minutes to establish relief and then lasts for 4 hours.

There are studies about all pain medications used in child birth around their efficacy. If you believe they only do good and trust your body to make sure they are safe for baby then that intention when strong enough is a very powerful force.

Remifentanil

This is fast acting and short living

Unknown influence on baby.

Epidural

A anaesthetic requiring a team of Anaesthetists which numbs the nerves that cary sensations from the birth canal to the brain.

This is delivered by a needle into the spine.

This may cause numbness in the legs.

Blood pressure changes and both you and baby will require constant monitoring so will be required in a hospital and are not available at home births. You can decide. Birthing babies advocates no particular position on pain relief. Your body your choice. We give you ways to be enough to birth baby with confidence and to reduce the sensation of pain with internal visualisation.

You being comfortable with your choices and your personal confidence and congruence is important and determining your intentions into life is the path of an empowered mother. The principle is state you intention and then determine it by persevering with that path with your full support and faith that that is right for you. So there is no judgement, no guilt but acceptance that this is the right path for you. When you own your choices you are much stronger. The journey that is just beginning.

Your partner can play an inclusive and active role in childbirth. Every step of the way. Through the journey of birthing babies and your experience of pregnancy and labour. Supporting you to support you to birth baby. You can begin to make your own list of what you require of your partner. In recent years separation was a key trauma for women who birthed through the pandemic and isolation conditions however with hope this time has passed. What would you expect from your partner what do you want from your partner. Below are suggestions. They are suggestions for you to build on. What are your expectations. With clear communication, you are building the role they will play through your labour from the very beginning. Then you can have the expectation of something good as labour begins.

PARTNERS ROLE

Perineal massage

Atmosphere of calm

Light touch massage - increase endorphins

Prompting techniques and
visualisations
With key words

Making informed decisions

Positive affirmations

Keeping the birth process
mother orientated by
leasing with care
professionals (your wishes)

Bonding with baby

"This aint over baby .... "

After birth, what to expect. Stage 4 the birthing of the placenta

At this stage you are bonding with baby. Precious moments that encourage the expulsion and sealing of the vessels in your uterus after the placenta is delivered

**MANTRA **

The vessels in my uterus close once the placenta comes away and my body can heal naturally.

My uterus is healing every minute with each breath I take the vessels are contacting and returning to their normal shape and role.

My body heals after birth with exceptional speed. My natural instincts now take over and heal my body with remarkable speed.

My body is instinctively programmed to heal while I occupy my time with attending to my baby.

The blood vessels in my uterus close firmly and the placenta comes away naturally there is no need for my body to retain it as it has served its purpose and can now be released.

As I tend my baby my body heals itself automatically with great speed so I can continue with my mission as mother with greater strength.

I am calm confident and in control as the final stages of labour are completed.
I am healing with each breath my body grows stronger
My baby is born strong and healthy.
My uterus can now heal and shrink back to its original shape and size with exceptional speed.

I am calm confident and in control.

Visualise the placenta leaving your body naturally on some occasions this may requires assistance once again you remain calm confident and in control as you do. After birth for this time as you are in your bubble with baby nothing else matters nothing matters. You are in the bubble of self love and the enjoyment of your baby being born.

You will feel the elation and joy of meeting baby for the first time.

The bond between you that has been growing through the past months the familiarity with your babies should their purpose intended by you and your purpose intended by you is now alive.

You are still one but together in a different way.

Now baby is here. Life is different and you can enjoy the flow of joy and happiness through each day.

Every day something wonderful happens such to remind me of the support of my world and the world around me.

As with every breath your sense of acceptance of the change can begin to become you.
Enjoy and become absorbed in every way with the future before you and the moments now of complete satisfaction that you and baby are well.
If at any time you require any assistance intervention you will remain calm confident and in control and intend for the health of your baby to take form and enjoy the sensations of meeting you baby for the first time
Seeing their tiny fingers and toes and its tiny fingers and toes and its features on its face its eyes as it looks at you.

Birthing babies has no particular position on intervention.
But only on the utilization of your natural ability to use your mind and body to reduce the likelihood of unnecessary intervention but if intervention is required then it is to be accepted and know that you fully support it to assist you in birthing baby safely.

Unnecessary intervention is different to necessary intervention.

And if you have required intervention to birth baby or chosen that path then that is also to be enjoyed as you still did it.

Women who are placed in the position of having elected caesareans to preserve baby can on occasion feel a Sense of failure that they did not do enough or did not do it properly in the pursuit of a natural birth.

There is no cause for the absolute determination on a natural birth to result in the feeling of failure if it is not achieved.

When your babies birth requires intervention it is a necessary endeavour however. What is important in the event of planned or unplanned c sections is the calibration of the differences of the natural hormones that are present in labour. When you don't labour baby the hormonal sequence is different so there is also an additional written session here to enhance the feelings of bonding with baby as if you had laboured.

The hormones that commence and prompt the forward flow of child birth are not present in a planned cesarean.

So in turn the recovery sequence the elation and the huge surge of oxytocin is not present so through relaxation and suggestion you can pre plan for this and make sure your emotional and internal nervous response can be aligned with similar sensations after the birth of baby even if you do not labour baby.

To encourage the release of hormones or mimic the sensations of the release of these hormones by suggestion to your body much the same as the desensitization to pain into discomfort you can turn the feeling of plannedness routine and anxiety into feelings of elation security and a sense of love as if oxytocin was the main component in the birth of baby.

So what do we have now.
Recap, so now you are pregnant. You know why, You definitely know how, and you have an understanding how hypnosis for child birth works, you have experienced it. You know about your body, it makes sense now, that relaxation isn't a huge ask at all, youre aware of the influence of your hormones and know how to work your nervous system in your favour at all times. Also The Love drug oxytocin is your best friend. And so are the ways to make it.... You know the science of fear, how to reduce it, You have the mental ways the physical ways and the environmental ways. You know how to influence your hormone balance and reduce stress hormones to the positive for the purpose you have for birthing babies. You know how to breathe, you know you have overcome many fears, and turned them into confidences. You know how to breathe, forever to bring you

calm. You have a confidence to prelude a c sections even if it is unplanned. You know how to increase your pain tolerance, to reduce discomfort. You know about mediation, you know you can make choices, and you know when labour is here what to do.

CHAPTER 6

" AFFIRMATIVE... CAPTAIN " ... WHAT YOUR MIND
CONCEIVES YOUR BODY CAN ACHIEVE.

POSITIVE AFFIRMATIONS FOR CHILD BIRTH

My babies birth will be incredible
An experience shared with my partner

Any fears belong to another space another place another time and irrelevant to the birth of this baby

My body was designed and built to birth this baby with ease.

I am relaxed and I am happy that my baby is about to be born.

Each contraction has a job to do – Once this contraction is complete I will never experience this contraction again.

I am looking forward to each contraction

I am working in partnership with my baby

As I am calm my baby will be so

As I am relaxed my body will birth my baby efficiently

My muscles work together by making birth easier

I relax as we move through each phase of birth as we work ta my bodies own pace

My body is working at its own pace

My body is positioned perfectly for each stage of labour

I will make decisions that are right for me and my baby

I am in tune with my body

I am in listening to the messages it keeps sending me

I will make decisions that are right for me and my baby

I am in tune with my body

I am working with the support I have around me.

I am supported within and around me.

I stay centred inside in my world as the world moves around me to birth my baby with ease

As change occurs within and around me I stay centred in the eye of the change I am strong, stable and always provided for.

After the birth of my baby My vessels contract and my placenta comes away easily after birthing my baby

I recover quickly and easily

What my mind conceives my body can achieve

As you appreciate now baby is here. You did it. Now the next chapter of your journey begins. Breathing into your life as a mother or a father or a parent.

As it sleeps the gentle rise and fall of babies chest as it breathes its first breaths independent of the womb and umbilical cord. I feel a sense of wonder and awe as I appreciate the miracle that is me and My newborn baby

You can become absorbed in the miracles of life and enjoy the moments in time fully present in adoration of baby and the your union with it. You birth together.

As you do your body will have comfort.

You can use everything you have learned to reduce the discomfort. Turn down the sensations of discomfort or pain or strain by using the dials.

Move slowly and frequently to ease the discomfort and move into healing.

**MANTRA **I am capable of birthing my baby with ease and confidence. I am a strong and confident woman. I am able, I am loved, I am supported by Life (the universe or your equivalent) within and around me. I am respected, appreciated, honoured. I am enough. I can support my baby fully. I am strong and always have and am enough to provide for me and my loved ones. I am balanced. I am centred. I am fulfilled each day in meaningful ways as a mother and a woman. I am confident of my ability to birth baby and be a extraordinary parent.

Recap, so now you are pregnant. You know why, You definitely know how, and you have an understanding how hypnosis for child birth works, you have experienced it. You know about your body, it makes sense now, that relaxation isnt a huge ask at all, youre aware of the influence of your hormones and know how to work your nervous system in your favour at all times. Also The Love drug oxytocin is your best friend. And so are the ways to make it.... You know the science of fear, how to reduce it, You have the mental ways the physical ways and the environmental ways. You knowhow to influence your hormone balance and reduce stress hormones to the positive for the purpose you have for birthing babies. you know how to breathe, you know how to You have overcome many fears, and turned them into confidences. You know how to breathe, forever to bring you calm. You have confidence to prelude a c sections even if its unplanned. You know how to increase your pain tolerance, to reduce discomfort. You know about mediation, you know you can make choices, and you know when labour is here what to do. You know how to mould your thoughts by using positive affirmations. You know how to communicate and encourage your partner to embrace your relationship and birth baby together as a team.

CHAPTER 7

" IT'S ALL ABOUT POSITIONING BABY "

"I am not Buddha. Rubbing my pregnant belly *will not bring you good luck, prosperity, or wealth." ...*

Strength in positioning

Traditionally we observe the birth giving position as laid on ones back, as this is what has been promoted in recent years. In the mainstream flow of the publicization and the publication of birth.

But it isn't how we are built to birth baby.

I t isn't how your body is designed to work nor is it how gravity works. Gravity is a powerful force and the above suggests we have been so possessed to ignore its influence in childbirth. One of the most powerful physical forces on the planet is there at our service ready and willing to support you in birthing your baby.

In birthing babies you are using every single natural asset you have.

When you look at the structure of the female form it's possible to appreciate its immaculate design. Every single cell has purpose and every single purpose has purpose. Every aspect of child birth is pronounced for by the immaculate development of the female form to make it so your body will present you with ways to reduce discomfort and more steadily reduce labour time by including (but not exclusively). Firstly your instincts will be louder to move when you feel the sense of discomfort. You will move and increase the movement and incidences of changing position. For centuries stretching yoga postures have been effective in relieving tension and some of the positions recommended are mirroring these traits when we feel pain the natural response is to curl into the pain rather than to stretch through the pain. It encourages constriction whereas a stretch and movement is a decompression and an expulsion of the energy of discomfort into a movement of the muscle in a way that makes sense to make good what is right. So the expulsion of the tension to move with the contraction is the endeavour. The constriction is the wave of motion bringing the baby out is the intention of the constriction the movement of your body in response to the constriction is to stretch rather than bend to the constriction. Awareness of the intention if the constriction is to move baby through like a wave of muscular movement.

And that movement is more effective without the contortion of your body with the pain. So the pain is the discomfort from the movement and your body will most naturally want to stretch to the pain to open the pathway for the contraction to fulfil it's purpose which is not to cause pain to you but to move baby down through the birth canal.

Positioning is to progress this. To progress the movement by enhancing your comfort and centering your intention in your body as a movement as well.

As centering your attention on movement is the purpose often distracted by the feeling or sensation of the pain labelling the movement and contraction of baby making its way down the birth canal. Birthing is a journey the original magical mystery tour. So the birthing journey for you includes the repositioning of your body, so as to respond to the contraction without constriction but to respond with opening and expulsion of the energy than notions you to bend into constriction with a stretch into comfort and relaxation led by your tension on calm confidence and in control. Birth is continuum a space and within this space you can trust your body and know that it know what to do. It is a day like no other and a day totally within your silent power.

BABYS EXPERIENCE OF BIRTH

Baby starts labour by producing hormones that start the production of oxytocin.
Baby wants to breathe that is reportedly what starts the process of labour.

ORIGINAL MAGICAL MYSTERY TOUR
The pressure builds around babies head (like putting a turtle neck sweater on.) Simultaneously the pressure is also building around the babies buttocks as the uterus contracts upon them and pushes baby along through the birth canal (very sensory like being hugged from all directions) Like a massage the muscles are massaging baby through the birth canal and as they do stimulating its innate systems of independent life support to life. Waking up, the heart lungs and massaging the skin for circulation walking baby into a independent life support where its body is able to thrive outside of the womb. The massaging stimulated the babies nervous system to excrete hormones and the chemical response required to thrive outside of the womb and this all happens while baby is moving through the birth canal into this world.

Massaging the skin and encouraging the cells to bring more energy to the surface of the body.

As you consider the baby has to the time been within its amniotic sac with very little contact and stimulation from outside of its body. It will now begin to wake up within the body to having an exterior. The sensation of closeness and contact being there. Being a comfort and being a now new continuum also.

The birth canal is 23cms long

As the babies crown reaches the pelvic floor muscles they are soft and springy and are eased over the head little by little massaging the Head up and down against firm resistance as baby crowns it head, Right angled bend babies head turns and its shoulders exit the birth canal into life.

BABIES EXPERIENCE OF LABOUR

Birth - breath - cry

Kicking reflex

Leads to nipple

Nourishment

Bond through scent - touch - sight and sounds

Tell your midwife you have used hypnosis for childbirth

POSITIONS FOR BIRTHING AND LABOUR

Purpose :
Enhancing the widening of the birth path
moving into comfort and shorten this phase of labour also
reducing likelihood of an episiotomy move your body gives
the energy of constriction and tension a means of expulsion
so you can turn the tension into calm using the meditations.
My vagina is relaxing to make way for the birth of my baby. My
cervix is relaxing and opening like a flower.
The muscles in my vagina are now relaxing and opening like
a flower to give the optimal opening for my baby to enter this
world.
I am calm confident and in control.
my vaginal walls are expanding in relaxation to allow the flow
of baby into this world. Combined with movement in stage
two labour this will influence your bodies ability to birth baby
with ease and facilitate faster healing after birth.

GROUPS EXERCISE PRACTICE ALL THESE
Practicing positioning through all stages of pregnancy will help and give you greater strength and flexibility in your whole body.

The more you use the positions the easier they will become when you need them, imagine the first time you use them is when you are 40 week pregnant in transitional labour the will likely be incredibly alien though when you use them life the audios as you are moving through this book make time. Use a journal to make space for you each day to prepare for birthing baby.

Leapfrog

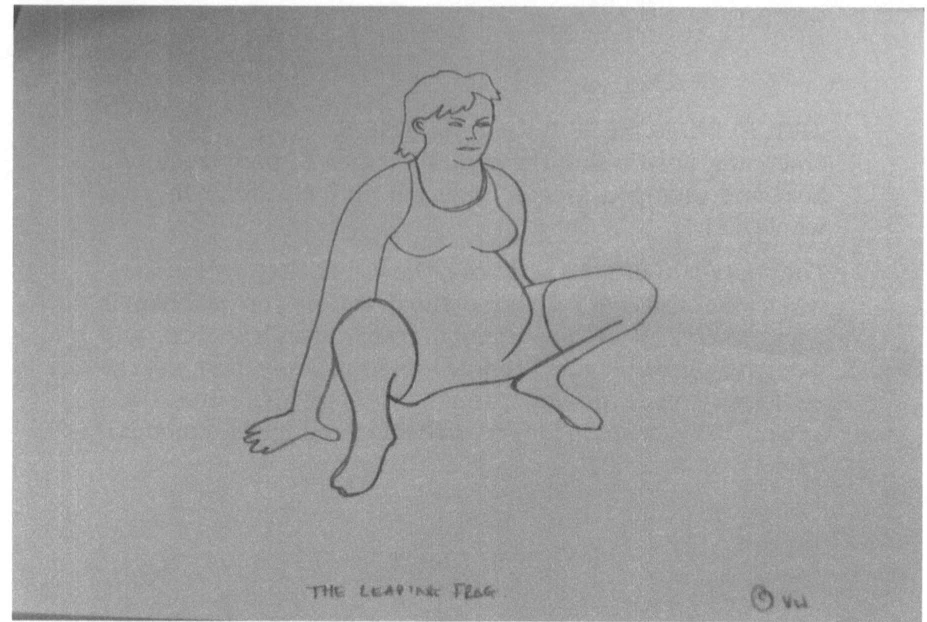

effects : opening of the pelvic region
reduced hip pain by stretching through
gives expansion to the shoulders and the back
relieves the constriction through stretching and requiring the energy of the body expand in to the spaces of movement where it will be naturally called to the places of the constriction or discomfort
Moves labour forward through is an effective redirection of your energy into calm movement and flow.
Practice strengthening your knees and ability to resume a stand when using this position while pregnancy progresses. So you build relative strength an balance. You will notice as you move through pregnancy your centre of balance shifts physically so, do this often.

Supported squat
For obvious reasons logistically - supported squat is helpful
benefits : the skin to skin contact from supporter reduces anxiety and stress hormones creating comfort.
Increases oxytocin production.
Stretches the posterior stretches discomfort through the back and also opening the pelvis and increasingly expelling tension turning into comfort

Bouncing in this position may also be helpful
pushing your back and pelvis down to release tension until
you are ready to push baby through the canal.

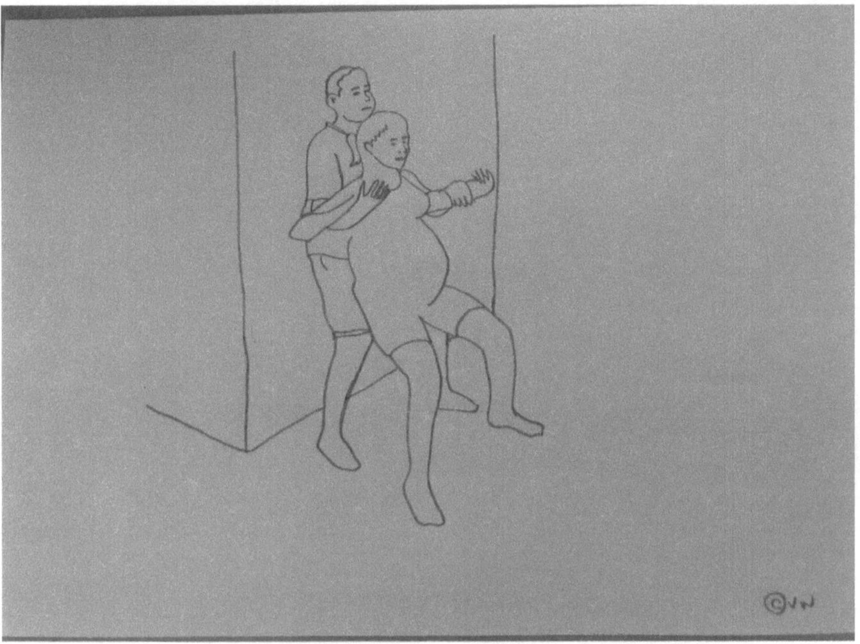

Hands and Knees
Reduces pressure on the back – spine and allows to stretch the
neck back and shoulders
Reduces pressure on the baby
Ensure knees and hands supported by pillows and someone
close to offer support incase of a sideways roll.

LEAPING FROG
POLAR BEAR

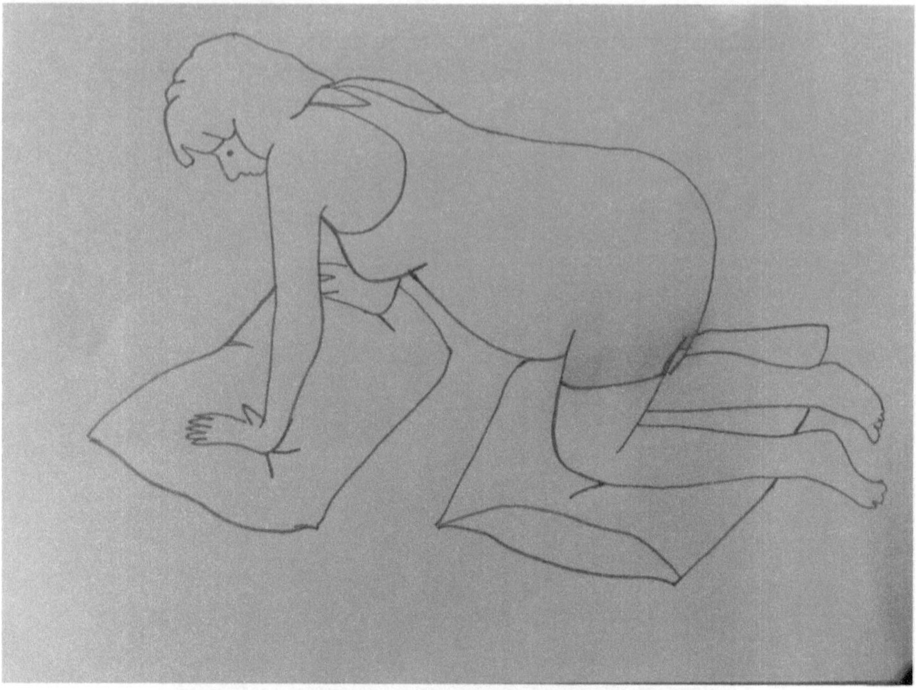

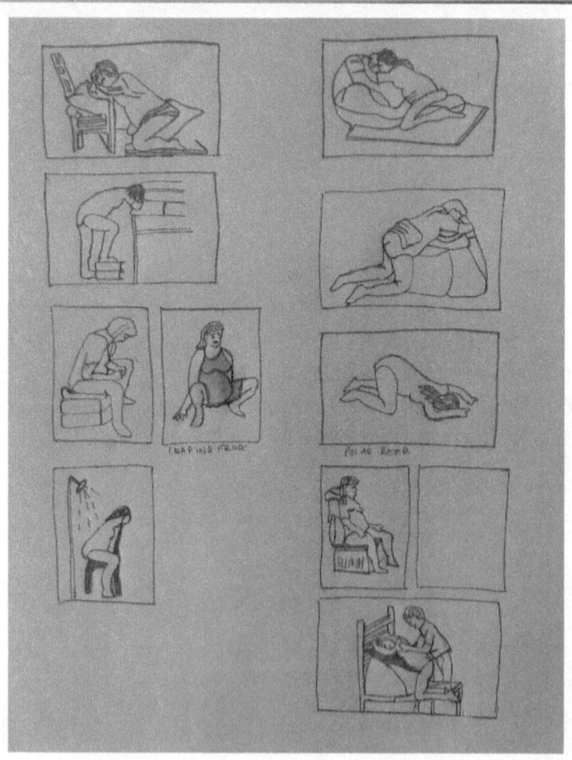

ADAPTED POSITIONS IN CONTEXT.

1 Knees to chair

Stretching back and encouraging gravity.

2. Elevated foot stretch – flexing the hips and allowing greater flow of energy through the pelvis region.

3. Shower – heat on your back and the sensation of water as a relaxation.

4. Reverse polar bear – useful in stage 2 breathing pushing baby down. Opens rib cage for air. Fully physically supported.

5.polar bear – bottom elevated – effective back stretch . Elongates the spine, to relieve tension and increase comfort.

6. CHAIR. Arms stretched behind chair to open rib cage and breathe more effectively. Opening up the rib cage and breathing tension into calm.

POSITIONING FOR EASE

benefits of each position

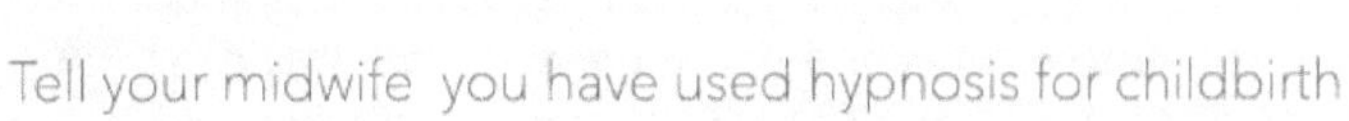

Position for the final stages of labour can be one of any. Depending on the position of baby the progression.

The aim: To preserve the energy you have and make childbirth most efficient
More efficient through breath
More efficient through movement.

Most efficient. Preserve the energy you have to progress the birth more quickly by remaining calm confident and in control.

You can now trust your body to guide you the appropriate position. You will know what is right for you.

Listening to your body and doing what is most comfortable for you.

What is most comfortable for you

As long as you do it with intention of health for you and baby then there can be no argument

You will find that you can nourish your body into recovery through eating rich fresh foods, vegetables and meat and fruit and you will be naturally guided to foods which will nourish you in the way your body requires nourishment for the coming weeks and months. Any excess that deplete you will be reminded to you by choosing more nourishing options so you can nourish your body for the coming weeks and months to prepare for the next chapter of childbirth and motherhood to a new born baby. During pregnancy using the positions and building a sense of familiarity with the positions makes them familiar. If you imagine just beginning to use them with a guide sheet when you reach labour thats not helpful. Don't be leaving this one to the last minute. Integrate these as part of your daily ritual.

When you reach the time for labour they will have become your natural lines to work into they will feel natural and they will serve the purpose of being a natural position in relieving the discomfort by the reasoning above. As you make time each week to use the positions your physical flexibility increases.

Recap, so now you are pregnant. You know why, You definitely know how, and you have an understanding how hypnosis for child birth works, you have experienced it. You know about your body, it makes sense now, that relaxation isn't a huge ask at all, youre aware of the influence of your hormones and know how to work your nervous system in your favour at all times. Also The Love drug oxytocin is your

best friend. And so are the ways to make it.... You know
the science of fear, how to reduce it, You have the mental
ways the physical ways and the environmental ways. You
knowhow to influence your hormone balance and reduce
stress hormones to the positive for the purpose you have for
birthing babies. You know how to breathe, you know how
to You have overcome many fears, and turned them into
confidences. You know how to breathe, forever to bring you
calm. You have confidence to prelude a c sections even if is
unplanned. You know how to increase your pain tolerance,
to reduce discomfort. You know about mediation, you know
you can make choices, and you know when labour is here
what to do. You know how to mould your thoughts by using
positive affirmations. You know how to communicate and
encourage your partner to embrace your relationship and
birth baby together as a team. you know how to position your
body for birthing. How to maximise the planetary forces to
assist you in birthing baby. You have a whole bunch of new
positions to add to your repertoire. And that is ok.

Next. It is all about envisioning the living.

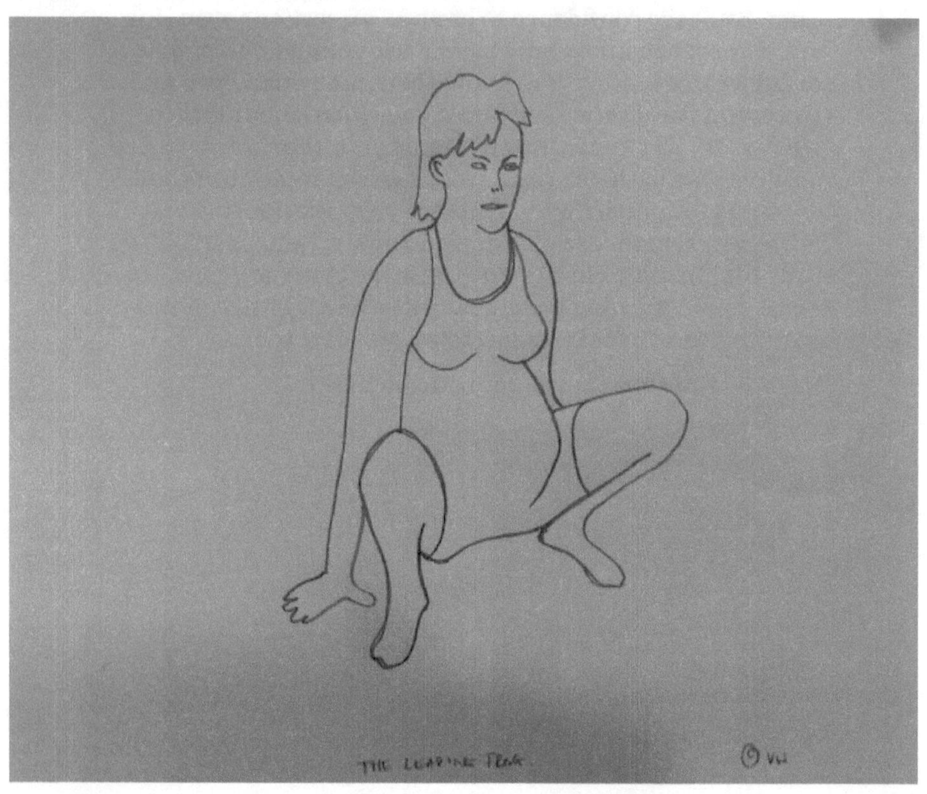

THE LEAPING FROG.

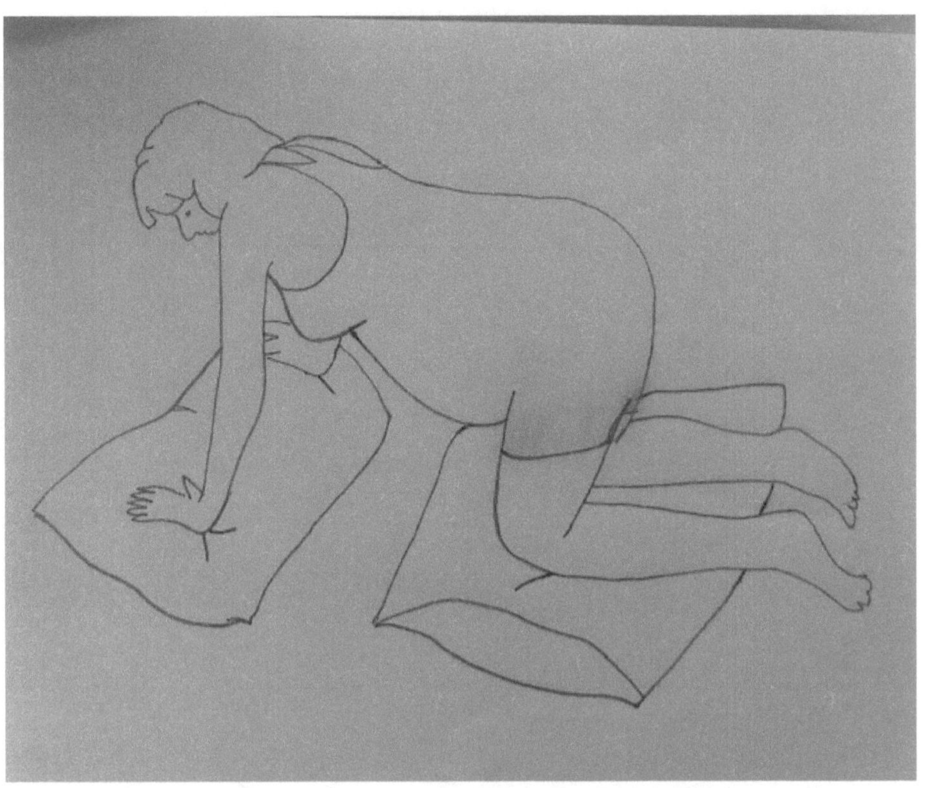

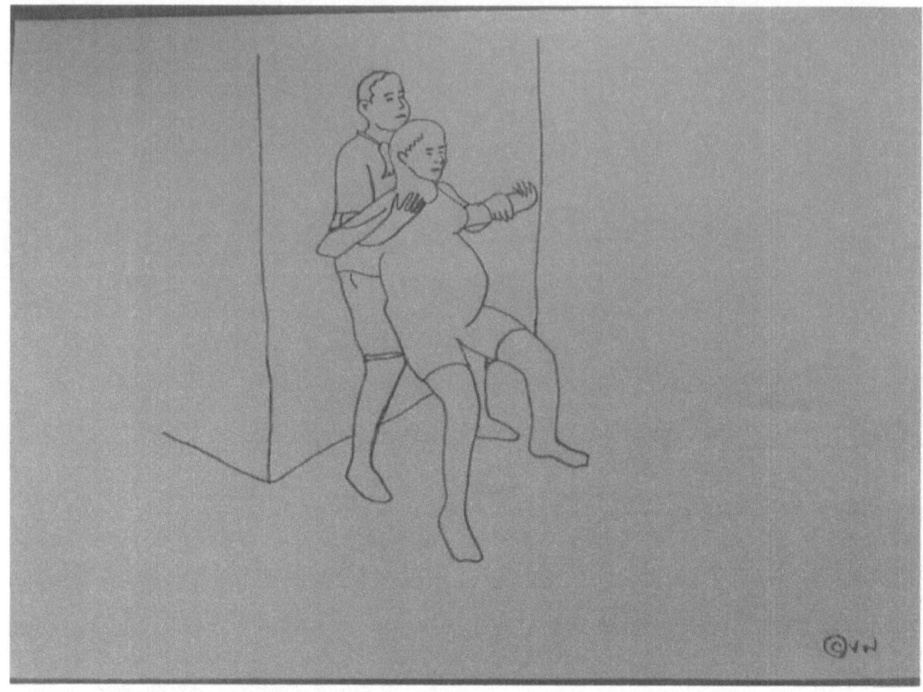

Child birth in Emergency

It is our response to emergent situations that is most important rather than the sudden and maybe totally unexpected situation with which we are confronted.
We have faced two world wars, Eastern conflict and unpredictable terorist activity, a global pandemic and natural disasters the list and variety of sudden traumatic events experienced in the lives of of us all goes on.

There is a quote from Marie Williamson

"Something very beautiful happens to people when their world has fallen apart: a humility, a nobility, a higher intelligence emerges at just the point when our knees hit the floor"

There is an insurmountable strength that rises in people when emergent situations occur. It is a calm that pervades all fear. A great composure that carries a person through situations. Until the danger or risk to life is averted. Love turns inward. Nothing else matters. Survival kicks in.

Nothing disturbs the more natural fear of child birth than fear. Fear disturbs the conscious and unconscious control of your natural process of fear. Love turns inward. You have experienced this in other situations you have experienced it in other contexts.

So when emergent situations occur within labour your are more rightly placed into composure using birthing babies techniques. Breathing and trusting that you are enough and the world your world will turn to support you.

CHAPTER 8

Post partum promise - Envisioning the living

"There are no words that can describe the euphoria you feel when your baby recognizes you for the first time and smiles."
—Jared Padalecki

"You are my sun, my moon, and all of my stars." — E.E. Cummings

Now the easy part is over you just have to keep it going. Allow the stars to serve you and reflect to you the mirror of your power to be a mother in the greatest sense. And Look what is ahead. Anything can change in a moment but right now you have a whole lifetime of future possibilities before you but you can also direct those possibilities you're your intentions. You choose.

Intentions held strongly enough direct your life. By the direction of your attention, is one way to move your life. To direct your attention with love and with the sense of feeling, is much more potent. So you can navigate changing circumstances within your own control and also direct the way they will become for you. And you can not only navigate what life brings but do so in choosing what life brings to you and navigate in such a way that your experience is your choosing. You can intend what you want and make it happen.

Not by force or will but by envisioning and tenacity and faith. Do this before the birth.

By intending what you want and setting those intentions to life before the birth, you are pre ordering a life to live when you really need everything you must keep you aligned moving forward. It's like someone preparing meals before the birth stocking your freezer with home cooked meals so they will be there when you are ready. It's the same principle. When you are tired and the long sleepless nights begin upon you. You will require something, something to bring you forward. When you are doing night feeds and when you feel like you want to give up give in and surrender to the something that is the easy way. Planning and preparing before birthing baby is so helpful because you are setting up your fall back for when you feel like you can't.

You are pre-loading your fall back so it becomes a fall forwards. When everything else is more important there you will be. Setting intentions before birth – because when hormones or healing are taking over, night feeds and tiredness. You still have the energy to honour these spaces. You have a plan. Also know when to ask for help with feeding, bonding, from partner, from others, communicate with the people around you about what you want, what you need and how they can support you in life. Doing this now will reduce the sense of post partum dips because you have engineered something to carry you forward. So you are reminded them you are reminded to your intentions. And you can make them move forward effortlessly. There will be a great pressure to do everything at once perfectly but Rome was built through time type of directive. Every day moving forward making progress.

First .... (The functional aspects) What's going to lower your energy

1.Doing it ALL

Night feeds and the intermittent rest periods do take
time to get used to. But you have a internal capacity
unknown to you at this time that will kick in when you

need it. To keep you going through these times.

When you are desperate to sleep and baby is feeding,"
it's only a matter of time " before the wound heals,
before the baby sleeps. before they stop crying before
you get to pee... before ... you fill in the blank .

One of the most powerful phrases during
the early months is this ....

" it is only a matter of time "

because there will be times when you feel like it is not going
to end the moment of discomfort. Of tension of crying
of ...... you fill the blank. But it does. And there is comfort.
When they are screaming it is not easy to Imagine the baby
sleeping. But imagine it. When they are crying it's not easy
to imagine them calm. Imagine it. Your intentions guide the
moment so being calm, and guiding the moment is helpful.

Breast feeding. Healing. Hormones. Diet. The company you
keep. Episiotomy and C incision site. Do you ever think when
you have a common cold, that you can't even remember how
it feels to feel normal, or well. Yes, that. Some say that each
cold is a healing so you will be stronger after it. Other times it
is just a similar sensation.

Just as all wounds will heal, it simply requires the focus
upon the healing and tightening beyond labour. You will
be encouraged to do pelvic floor exercises to resume the
strengthening of the muscles which have been used within
pregnancy, and any lesions healing. As well as your body you
can use your mind to direct the healing of your body after
child birth. The most important thing is to stay centred and
be gentle with yourself. You imagine beyond birth, wounds
healing wound tightening of the pelvic floor strengthen
each day, healing cleanly fresh new skin and muscle and
a cooling ocean wave like sensation of water flowing over
any areas of heat or soreness. Intend they strengthen and
minimal scaring, healing the skin perfectly and the muscles
being brought together perfectly and merging and meshing

into a comfortable and tight form with maintained sensation and all of the pleasures you can enjoy from normal every day acts and even intimacy being increased and sensations maintained. This being your intention it will guide you actions. Tightening muscles doing repeated exercise, little by little. But repeated exercise will in turn bring strength. For example, The nerves, that carry the impulses are like roads see them growing back perfectly flowing traffic, for pleasure and sensation to return. Each time building a sense of trust and faith and desire without the fear of discomfort you can induce the greatest sexual experiences by moving very slowly. So that when you are fully sexually active again you will feel ultimate pleasure. Any traces of traumatic memory can be re-laid using the idea that they can be re-laid as pleasure paths now can replace the other paths creating new pathways of pleasure becoming possible so the sensation will be returned as is perfect and the pleasure centres reformed and strengthened so you can enjoy great pleasure beyond the birth of baby. This can become a mantra and visualisation. Everything coming together. Everything is coming together.

It really is possible to influence this within your mind. I can now fully experience the pleasure of intimacy.... and (you can expand with your personal wishes and desires.) Holding onto any traumatic memory may reduce the healing in your body. Using visualisations will help. Using birthing babies every technique through labour will increase the possibility of your birth being experience being one where you are calm confident and in control. One that you positively remember Using confident birthing. The dials, The candle layers, The beach meditation.And rejuvenate. They are adaptable and will give you new ways of overcoming all the small challenges that come in the early days postpartum. They will keep working in new ways to open new solutions new channels. Each transferable in perspective in life. All in sequence strengthen so many aspects of your unconscious ability to birth your baby in a way that preserves the perfection and integrity of your physical body enables it to birth with minimal strain and also enables you to heal more effectively and facilitate natural processes such as feeding by visualizing the flowing of milk in your milk ducts imagine. Breathe in cool breathe out the heat breathe in cool.

2. Intimate care

Using the toilet after any surgical intervention to your perineum may incite fear instinctively in the body. Remain Calm. Cool and calm, ice packs, and visualising cool water flowing and the colour blue bringing the sensation of cool (practical additions for healing - Imagine ...Cool and calm cool and calm and then be sure to rinse with warm salt water on each occasion dry thoroughly when you urinate) So again when you poo. You may need to push and use muscles you have worked through labour. The visualisation for smooth flowing and a helpful fixation alternative – imagine a river flowing a stream and logs flowing through the river with ease and comfort they will flow through a small opening a under a small bridge without obstruction just flowing easily and comfortably through the opening. And intend this directed towards your abdomen while you are on the toilet and it should help; Each muscle relaxing comfortably to enable the logs to pass through the bridge very comfortably and smoothly – repeat repeat. It is so simple. But so effective.

Vaginal healing, my vaginal muscles are growing tighter and tighter every day. As they relaxed to allow for the birth of my baby they can now tighten with great comfort and ease. each and every day growing tighter and more toned, healing any scars or wounds to their pre pregnancy tension.

3. Breasts

Calming milk ducts imagine them as if they are two mountains and imagine there are many streams. If you are experiencing them as volcanos, use your minds eye to turn them into lush green mountain, flowing rivers a tributaries, cool and calm as the river in your mind flows freely cool and calm and soothing, bringing rich lush green calm growth to these areas. Until you can no longer visualise them as vulcanos and see them only as rich lush flowing rivers through lush green topped mountains and they will soothe. Repeatedly visualising, you will find that they become more

calm. The simple imagination of and visualization repeatedly
will have only positive benefits.

Nipples dry and cracked. With your nipples in mind, imagine
a desert plane as that the current state then imagine the
rain fall, soothing cooling calming rain fall. And the cracks
in the desert floor disappearing into streams and lush green
growth, fresh growth calming and soothing as streams
run through where the desert floor is now lush and green
and rejuvenated, cool and calm. You can feel the rush of
the gentle breeze and a wave a cool calm washing over you.
Imagine the cool calm water of the stream as if it is running
through your body and feel the sense of calm on your breasts.
Cool and calm flow. Cool and Calm. Repeatedly using this
visualisation and expand with your own imagination....
Your own ideas. Calming sensations cooling visualisation
(ice pads) Repeating these visualisations will bring comfort.
Through time even immediately. Especially when you have
the post natal anxiety and the mother baby cord pulling
from outside rather than inside. We don't consider it before
they are born, but when my son was born, I was a hundred
mile a minute woman who did everything, infallible. Sat
there in the hospital alone, with my son, it dawned on me for
the very first time. They cry, we immediately feel it. They
move and you feel it. Something so small as needing a wee.
There was no one to ask for help, so we went together. That
can overwhelm you if you let it. And for the first time, it
dawned on me, that now they are outside it's different. You
are with them all of the time. In a different way. You have to
protect them from the world outside. The dawning of the
responsibility and tie was huge. But it was mine, alone to
carry. And still is. I love it it's one of my greatest joys. Never
let that pressure drown you. Keep swimming, keep breathing
and definitely keep your head above the water. Because there
is always, time to breathe and be alone, always time to restore,
reset. Always enough of you. It is just about planning. Making
time for you no metter how short that is. (obviously do
consult with a medical professional alongside these advices if
you feel low, or have symptoms of PND).

Encouraging milk flow, imagine lush green abundant growth
in the Alveoli plenty fresh reservoirs always full and ready
to nourish and flow through tributaries like a linked river

system perfectly formed to assure the flow of the river of life giving fluid through these branches through the ductulus and ducts to the nipple and then flowing through ... adaptions on this theme and making your own visualisations is really effective. You can visualise it. Calming volcanos for eruptions... as simple as it sounds this is the language your body speaks and needs you to use..

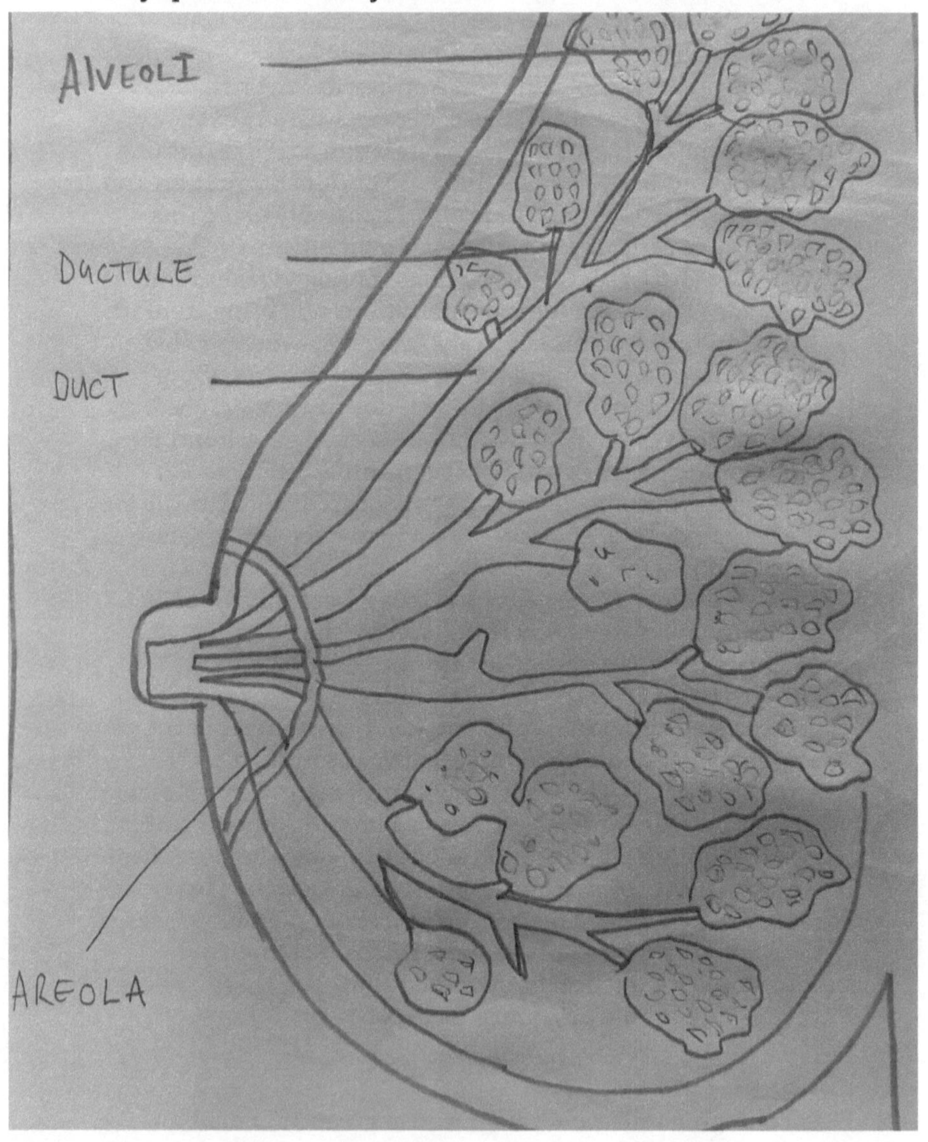

4. Self care. Nourishment. Managing your energy. Hormones.

Your hormones will fluctuate. It's a certainty. The one way you can influence this, is by knowing being aware that it will happen. Then you wont feel that something is not working or interpret it as if you are failing etc etc When your hormones change your perceptual filters may shift. But that's what it is, a similar sort shift as PMS. You may want to cry, laugh, throw something. Accept it as what it is. Youre still ok. You will feel different. And that's ok.

You can prioritise making time when it feels there is none to Nourish you. In whatever way you need, some women will crave mental nourishment and miss the activity and conversation, social aspects of work, others will miss the sense of themselves that was, whatever your nourishment requirement is you will have one so feed it. Little by little day by day. Your world is baby, and there is still time for you. So when you plan for it there is no internal war. Because it's there already. What is your nourishment. Nourish your intellect nourish your body nourish your self. Everything that you put in your body is wholesome. It might not be. What your head is craving. Because there is a likelihood you will crave something instant. Instant food or instant mental attraction. Mentally a pod cast, something to alert your senses. Fast energy. In the moments of tiredness moments of sadness or emotional fluctuation. When you just need something NOW. You reach for something nourishing. We generally hear these signals as a need for food, Quick food fast food, and sugar highs. But quite often its our mind needing something, not food, stimulation, a kind word, encouragement a hug, a pep talk or just a moment. So be sure not to confuse the two. And re balance your instincts so you begin to become attuned to the fact that this nourishment is more beneficial and more calming more wholesome and more steadying which is what you require in these times.

Your greatest line of defence against post natal dips and periods of depression is to make sure you eat well and stay focused forward. Nourish your body and mind. Coffee is a good perk up. Sustained by a wholesome snack. Comparison. Were looking towards granola rather than a can of Monster.

Like quick hits in life – easy come easy go. You want

something that sticks. Envisioning the living Is the organic oats, wholesome and fulfilling and the innocent smoothie, fresh salad of your life making sure you have the sustainable ability to move forward beyond the next emotional high into another phase. From high to low unlike a yo yo, but with a set point centrally and the ability to wind your self back in. Sustainable maintenance and the highs and lows, but make sure you have your central calibration, or set point to swing from and to. And make sure it someplace that's nourished, fulfilled inside. (as much as you can be with a new-born baby) We have highs and lows but it is so much better for your body when you can sustain a calm centre point. You can sustain this and that is easy. Rather than the instant wins and the highs and lows a sustainable setpoint, which is consistent enough to take the highs and the lows and still keep you winning with the strength for growth is really important within your self. Laying long term intentions, then suitably fertilising them with your attention, consistently. Every day so something. Whilst returning inside to your setpoint. One way you can ensure your mental health post partum is to make sure you avoid as many of the highs and lows as you can, they will happen, night feeds, long nights, isolation, loneliness. Generating sustainable energy.

When you are strong enough introduce light exercise gentle weights 1kg + so you can do them even when your feeding baby. Leg lifts while sitting raise a leg repeatedly. Each action will build muscle and strength, build stamina, increase your blood flow. Give you a general feeling of greater health. And your strength. When you hold more muscle, you hve greater energy reserves. Gentle day by day building.

Making sure you have a centre point that is calm and balanced. That will sustain you through time. And keep your emotions on an even keel. Your body will crave something to nourish it. So as your mind calms and is redirected by your forward facing intentions your body and mind begin to work together in harmony. You have the capacity to experience both and both has value so you can choose which is right for you in the moment.

In a different context. Sustaining your energy over time and having short burst of great activity or energy bursts. Book vs Podcast. Coffee vs water. Run vs walk. During postpartum promise you will be balancing the two. But they are not to content each other. Balancing rest and play - uptime and

down time much as babies rhythm. And this you can do then you are in harmony with baby and harmony with yourself.
In alternate context you have Expansion periods of great activity and then rest time for restorative purposes. Spend time around people who make you feel good.

What is your nourishment.

Nourish your intellect, nourish your body nourish your self. Everything that you put in your body is wholesome. It might not be. What your head is craving. Because there is a likelihood you will crave something instant. Instant food or instant mental attraction. Mentally a pod cast, something to alert your senses. Fast energy. In the moments of tiredness moments of sadness or emotional fluctuation. When you just need something NOW. You reach for something nourishing. I repeat this because it is important. We generally hear these signals as a need for food, Quick food fast food, and sugar highs, but quite often it is our mind needing something which isn't always food related. So be sure not to confuse the two. And re balance your instincts so you begin to become attuned to the fact that this nourishment is more beneficial and more calming more wholesome and more steadying which is what you require in these times. Your greatest line of defence against post natal dips and periods of depression is to make sure you eat well and stay focused forward. Nourish your body and mind and have hope.

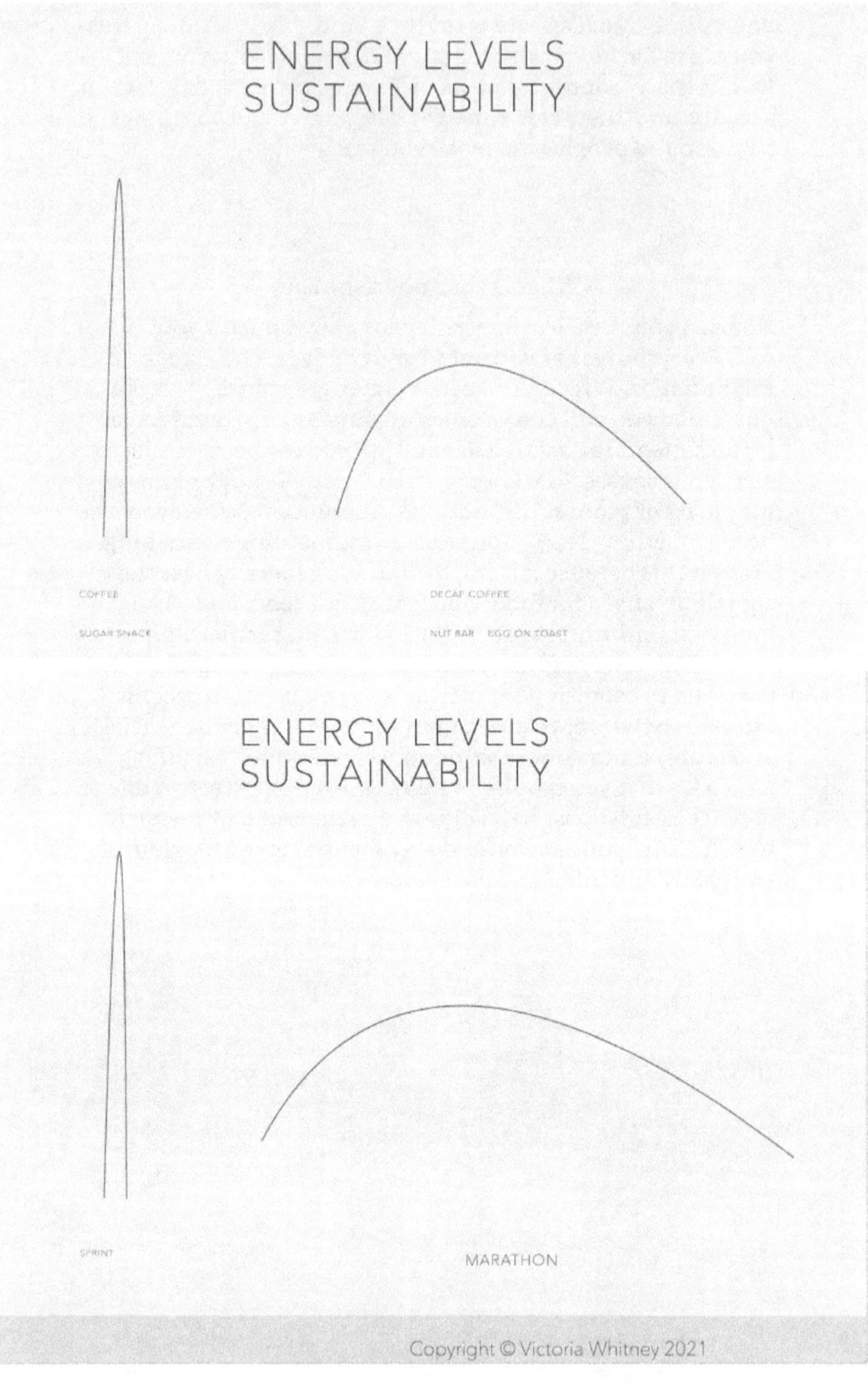
ENERGY LEVELS
SUSTAINABILITY
COFFEE
DECAF COFFEE
SUGAR SNACK
NUT BAR   EGG ON TOAST
ENERGY LEVELS
SUSTAINABILITY
SPRINT
MARATHON
Copyright © Victoria Whitney 2021

In a different context. Sustaining your energy over time and having short burst of great activity or energy bursts. Book vs Podcast. Coffee vs water. Run vs walk. During postpartum promise you will be balancing the two. They begin to complement each other. Balancing rest and play - uptime and down time much as babies rhythm. And this you can do then you are in harmony with baby and harmony with yourself. You know when they say that women who live in the same households menstrual cycles seem to align so they all menstruate at the same time. It is like that. You will at some point lead your cycle out though. Because baby will eventually go through the night. The key is to maintain your energy by short bursts and prolonged activity. But to return to a baseline, or set point.

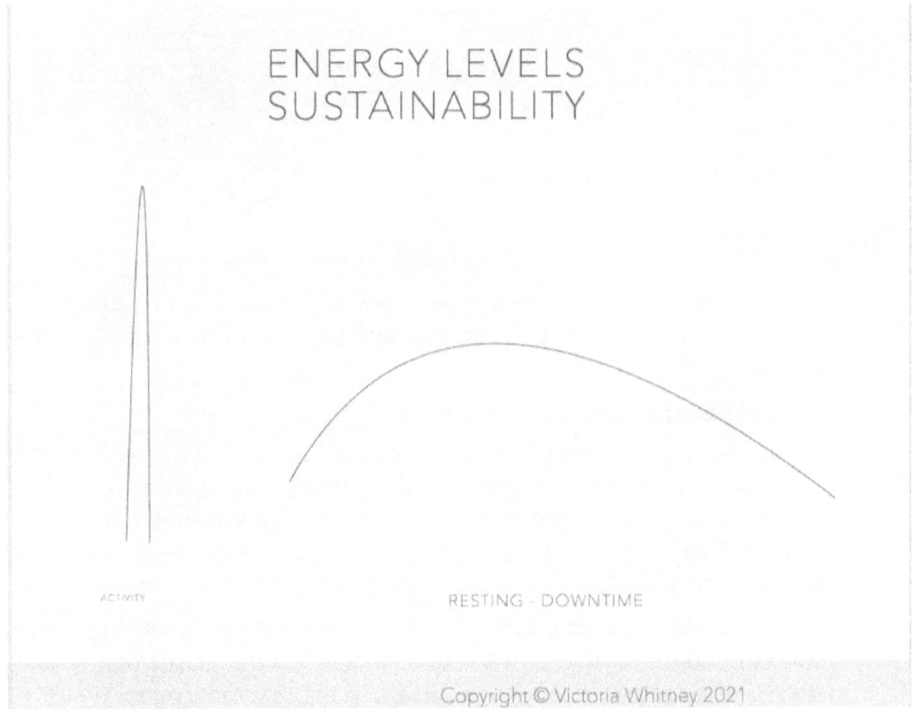

In alternate context you have Expansion periods of great activity and then rest time for restorative purposes.

ENERGY LEVELS
SUSTAINABILITY

All have value, But you choose how your balance sits. Just by thinking about it can start to reevaluate your own natural cycles.

Each cycle is present in everyday life.

To be aware of these so you can make sure you rest restore your body mind and soul building at the same time as sustaining. By including something that nourishes and sustains you in the finite capsules of time that will be available to you. Because you are always working towards the

greater vision. You can rest but you are always purposefully working towards the greater vision. You might gain great nourishment from doing the household chores, making sure the house is tidy or you might gian nourishment from a walk in the woods or a workout at home, or relaxation sessions, even lighting a candle, tending to some plants it may feel like the most non-sensicle thing to do because this needs doing and this needs doing and so does this. Appreciation is essential, appreciation of you and all that you are. When you are giving allot of you attention to everything else which is natural in early motherhood days. Take a moment. Even if it is just a moment - 10 minutes a day to work on your forward vision. Centre on something and to regain your core central balance that is wise calm and collected. By being fully aware of the moment as well as the " have to's " But growing the sensation for the moment and carrying that within you as you nourish everything else as well. Turn the have to's into Love to's. So you are always moving with love. There are time in the early days when you may have movements when you feel like you are disappearing ... that who you were is changing it isn't. These moments will encourage your essence to remain within you and your love and appreciate be relived with in you rejuvenating you and your sparkle as well as your overwhelming love for baby. You also have your overwhelming love for you and all that is important to you.

Feeding

Feeding Primary breast isn't always best – you are enough even if you choose formula or choose to change from breast to bottle. So commonly a point of angst so lets look it over, so you are bullet proof. Your choice once again will be the right one. Be forgiving of yourself and show yourself compassion. The pressure on this point is often great. But it is not. The priority is that your baby is nourished. That they are growing. That they are healthy. The relationship between that and your ability to breast feed is different. You are forgiving of yourself if breast feeding does not become so easy for you. Birthing babies has no position on which is best. But we do acknowledge the woman who thinks for one second that she is less than because she did not breast feed. The real question is was your baby fed and nourished. Yes. Then you have succeeded.

What is best for you, for your baby and your life circumstances, no judgement can be made equivocally scientifically, which is best. When I studied psychology in 1996 in each and every situation there is the nature nurture debate. What's innate and what is learned – then the interactionist position which is akin to sitting on the fence but it's an appreciation of both aspects with the ability to identify the relationship between the two. And balance that. In most circumstance dependent on the other variables. Science works in a controlled environment where everything is controlled. When in life there are so many outlying variables to form a judgement based on someone else's norm. It isn't either one. Nor a stance to use to punish oneself with feelings or thoughts of failure because they chose either way, nor is it to be a yardstick for someone else to take that stance upon or around you to influence you by pressure. It just is what it is, so as long as you own your choice, you can proudly live it. You know inside what is right for you and bearing in mind you have carried baby in your womb for 40 weeks there is a sense of familiarity that no one can challenge. You will know what is best. The feeding regime and choices should be made up balanced on research, and your own choices an your instinct being an integral part of that. Your own ideals and once again if there is a reason you can't then that is ok. If you desperately want to breast feed seek advice from your midwife and use all the techniques, if you have done everything and it is time to move to bottle. Then know you have done all that you can. Accept the priority is that baby is nourished. Then you have succeeded.

Your Sense of what is right for both you and baby, once again will reign. Because if it doesn't feel right to you it is likely there is a Reason why.

What Sustains You

Your Mainstay

Your rock, Your core your vision your unequivocal loves and your vision moving forwards.

When I say this it may be your partner it may be your children your career, some other external form of identity which is great value to you, but there are more, there are your aspirations. There are your character essences and strengths that will be reflected in your career your relationships, home and anywhere else you look because they are you. They are your strengths characteristics and everything you are mirrored in your world. You can strengthen them, when you accept, and acknowledge them.

What sustains you nourishes you keeps you centred. When the pulls on your attention are so great, what is your mainstay that holds in the centre of your world. That holds your world to you. What is your central focus. Your you ness. That sustains you. When you are reminded to it you can embody it when you need. It can be a vision of how you want things to be.

Next, State your intentions.

This doesn't need to be a struggle. Sometimes to ask people what they actually want in life, their face turns white and they start twitching. They have never been asked before. So take your time think about it. It does need to be concise. It helps to mould how you assert your time your intentions. You daily focus. Your intentions become reality so to make it concise enables you to realise what it was you were intending to do before you begin upon it. When you state your intentions.They keep you in check. Allot of the times we perceive a need for external accountability but often it is actually an ability we possess of our own. You know what is right for you the more you listen inside. When the external clutter is quiet you can listen not to a sound or a voice but a rhythm. A rhythm that is yours. It's your own heart beat and how it transpires in your life is unique to you but it is there when you hear it you can intend more clearly. It comes from the silence. The shusshing of our internal dialogue, just by being calm and aware, and gifting yourself the time and space to be, to breathe. To hear you. Allow aside the static, like the noise, and make sure your intentions are pure without judgement " on the others " what is it that YOU want. Just move with pure intent. The stuff is just stuff. It's unnecessary. Troublesome When our motivation is moulded by past experiences it is less helpful. Overcoming many of the fears and associations you have with motherhood so far in this book your perception is different. So the more you move with the love of birthing baby and its eternal innate bind of maternal love, On the whole your intentions will be founded in love. And love is a powerful thing. Balance listening to your instincts an distilling what you intend to the future Distilling refining it's a refinement process. Stripping away the unnecessary thoughts fears, intentions, and directions. "The stuffs " for example. The non sentimental loudness of the media, of the opinions. As you grow your listening you will find they begin to roll of your space, your aura or hue you create by strengthening the self, like Water of a ducks back. It is like some people when you look at them, have a jaggedy hue of noise. While others have a hue of " perfection" You aim for the latter. It is smoother and really does feel better. In this age there is allot of nose, noise is good, it has purpose but there are times just like the ebb and flow of the tide and the cycles of the moon when there is a space for stillness inside. The noise. That is what attracts and makes people look to it. It's intended to make noise so people follow. But it is always the same.

There is time to make space for still ness inside so you can intend. This doesn't always need to be a military operation to being about this time. Perhaps a walk in the park with a note book or even a moment, making a vision board. The people will not change but the intention you have will be stronger because your motive and intention is pure. So there will be less noise. You listen to you as much as the noise. And then suddenly the noise becomes less consuming. Once you intend and state your intentions you have direction you have direction and purpose. So the noise is less appealing and less heightening. Your purpose is quiet. Even if spoken to no one – in fact when it silent it is more potent because the sentiment of it remains within you. And moves you without a word. As intended by you for you. Without assumption that there you are within a partnership. Either with another or with yourself.

 A note to the single parents, You have strengths you had not even realized you had. You have more room in you to make a future plan for life and anything really is possible. More than often it seems like the reflection of others in partnerships, is defeating, like there is a presupposed something missing because of the logistical variables that are effective for single parents. But you can become more savvy, smarter, sharper in your instincts. No weaknesses only strengths. Anything is possible. As if it had been intended rather than had happened to you or upon you because now in this process you get to choose and make what you choose to happen, happen. Choose to change it by accepting w perhaps it was meant to be for now and the next chapter is what is important. During your whole pregnancy, building up to birthing, you grew a baby inside with no real thought your unconscious mind, and your body just did it. Now you can do the same with life. Take the time to intend for you. Some people call them goals – Goals are outdated. But intentions and experience become real. It all sounds very velveteen rabbit. But I'm a huge believer in this. Having moved through the goal setting era I find intentions and determination make the things happen, because it's the process unbranded. DE Jargoned but a real actual process of the doing to make the having. Intentions, are visions, intended to be lived. The real life living of the intentions you determine into living experiences that are intended to be lived by you. Goals can be moved. But when you are intending with deliberation. Things happen.

Living the vision

The FUTURE IS YOURS
Make a plan
Write that sh*t Down
work on it
every
single
day

So reflecting to the past. When something has been that was not your choosing. For whatever reason. It just wasn't the time. Now is the time.
You. Are. Enough. You have enough within you, you have strengths you had not even realized you had. You have more room in you to make a future plan for life and you have the most potential because you are here now. In truth it will be what you think of it , so believing that you have the capacity to hold enough and are always becoming more, and once again everything you need and want is always provided for you in some way will take you a long way. Your instincts

will support you and the more you respect and love your self, the more you will be found into what is right for you. As if it had been intended because you chose it. You get to choose and make what you choose to happen, happen. During your whole pregnancy, building up to birthing, you grew a baby inside with no real thought your unconscious mind, and your body just did it. Now you can do the same with life. Take the time to intend for you. Some people call them goals – Goals are outdated. But intentions and experience become real. It all sounds very velveteen rabbit. I'm a huge believer in this. Having moved through the goal setting era I find intentions and determination make the things happen, because it is the process unbranded. DeJargoned but a real actual process of the doing to make the having. Intention are visions, intended to be lived. The real life living of the intentions you determine into living experiences that are lived by you.

Because if you do not define it then others will define you.

BEYOND BIRTHING THE FUTURE IS YOURS

Setting the space for your future- vision boarding

Defining what you want for your family

Vision Boarding takes moments - But it is in your awareness very day. Growing and becoming.

Money - I was toying and set an intention to make £4000 in

the space of 1 week.

I listed all the things I wanted the money for and all the ways I could make instant cash right now.

Then I forgot.

I woke up went about my day and things started to change …

When you state intentions and become your own accountability you are Making this automatic.

A few examples of how intention works. When your intention is concise. A couple of years ago …. And I was staying in London, I had driven through the night went straight to training, walked home to my hotel… for the entire day the hotel had been without electricity … The exact moment I approached the desk the lights came on the computers started working so I could check in to my room. Things like this happen when you work on your self. When you trust and move forward doors will open. Example two When you need to get moving … I was living in a small bungalow I thought had the great idea to downsize then have another baby …

A mother, baby is 6 months old and I'm at home hoping for something to change …. Half believing it wouldn't. Everything that was making it not possible was right there for me everything that was right all the reasons all the excuses all the …. STUFF .

So one day I just woke up with a fierce f 'this shit I want things different sort of feeling. I looked out of my window and said to my inner mind. What do you want to see when you look out of the window. " Project green fields "as my view. Exact words.

Then my then fiancé came home. We had a look. There it was. It has green fields panoramic to the front elevation Open sea views on three sides. And it was double the size of the previous house and within budget. We viewed and within 8 weeks we moved in. I am still here.

Back to this one... Money - I was toying and set an intention to make £4000 in the space of 1 week.

I listed all the things I wanted the money for and all the ways I could make instant cash right now.

Then I forgot.

 I woke up went about my day and things started to change ...

Within 14 days - I have upgraded my car £2500 cash

Received a cheque in the post for £1000 - The thing is they were known ways that just happened to be called in at the time when I intended.

And had new bookings in my business .

 A bump of just over £ 4000...

It is possible to make sudden and rapid changes and it is also possible to sustain this over time steady and slow and rapid change. It all depends how fierce you intend and for the time around birth you will require a gentle approach, because you require balance, and nourishment, but with the ability to make rapid change should you so need.

 Look at each space in your life individually. Health – body healing / shape eg Career – making this work with baby Home – now and progression next steps Family and relationship – your partner and strengthening your commitment. The early years can be a time of great happiness but also great challenge on the partnership. Make sure yours is bullet proof and that you share the acknowledgement that you are a team equal in ways. Work together as increasingly these are the relationships that hold. They tend to be constricted when one or other of the partners does not feel supported. But much like labouring and strength in positioning this is transferable, ideology stretch out the tensions make sure your relationship bends and moves with the transitions of parent hood as well. Is mutual flow and Communication, time for each other and baby, mutual love and support and trust. Oftentimes when one partner is weak the other raises to meet the bar. And that does not mean go to the pub.

The things you love most about life and increasing the amount of them that you experience. List them vision board them do whatever you need to keep them as a focus in your day. The more you do this you, and make sure you will have everything you really desire. Again when the temptation arises to settle to downgrade don't compromise, like reaching for a sugar snack when you could have something really nourishing. Like impulse buying and the regretting it later. And come form a place of not enoughness. These are your commitments to you for the next transition in life. They are defining moments and what you believe you extend and the mirror of you life will return to you opportunities in alignment with this. It sounds like a tough path. Though it isn't it is simply a path carefully and attentively trodden. You walk with care through the pathways of your life. Setting this now is Inoculating you around sleepless nights night feeds pressures of money etc etc There will be days but these underlying intentions are so much greater than the other else that is spinning around you. There are going to be moments when you feel like you are pushed to the very extreme so you Set your inner cheerleader dialogue now. By appreciating your great strengths and appreciating who you are. So when those moments come, which they will when you have very little to spare and have somewhere inside you know where to look to where you are all of these things and more. You have more emotional sustenance and stamina. Play the long game. Hold out for what is right.

Holding your best you

I am…..

I am…..

I am…..

I am…..

I am…..

I am…..

I am…..

WHEN YOUR SELF TALK ISN'T LEADING YOUR CHEERS.
A REMINDER FOR YOUR INNER CHEERLEADER

You stay centred in the eye of the change and know that love is stable and always provides for you and your loved ones. Is a powerful prayer. Even when it sounds innocuous. This resonance will overcome any obstacle. Reassurance that everything will be provided that you are more, have more always Everyone else may be really " helpful " And share wise words based on their own experiences. But your intentions are to be honoured, You have a clear space and time where you can move your intentions forward if you determine them enough. I always induce my clients, to manifest a bubble of consciousness within and around themselves. Such that they have the strength for well meaning comments that are not in alignment with their highest and best wishes for themselves, so they wash over them like water of a ducks back. Such that they can politely make and assert the intentions and actions which strengthen their purpose. With great strength and diplomacy. So you can move your world with you intention in a kind, gentle and diplomatic way. As well as with great force and strength. Blessed with advice from family and friends which you should choose to take accept modify is your own choice your own will and will be completely ok.

Always having the intention you do what is best for your vision of you and your family moving forward. Which can be enhanced yet untainted by the opinions of others unless they support you. Solution for the highest good always be guided to what is right for you. Even the small things, right instinct right shop right park right place at right time for the solution to flow. Building beliefs that draw the intended, and deflect the alternative. Because you never settle. More so how do you do this. You make new rules. Each day make a 10 minute time frame to note. 10 successes 10 things you are grateful for. Acknowledge 10 things you love. Embellish your day with some kind of celebration of what you do and who you are. Make that your routine. No matter what the day has entailed.Every Day. So they go noticed. Never lost beneath the noise.

You build a sense of cohesion from consistency. You will gain a certain clarity. Whether something is a yes or a no, you will have a sense of cohesion beyond birth that builds as you take these very simple steps. To avoid post natal dips. And make sure every day you do something for you. This is how you build your inner strength and perseverance. Each day these small acts become greater. You are strengthening and that requires that you make acknowledgement of your personal assets of character. Your inner cheerleader. That you Have about you that will give you the invisible   force field, a field around you anything that is counter to what you believe will simply roll off like water of a ducks back. This is your unwavering faith is built by daily acts that confirm to you your priority and that is you and the way you intend with each and every act each and every thought and each and every moment. That's mindfulness. It's silent. intention is silent. We can speak it but when you hold it inside, it builds. Having a plan and at the same time Letting go of the plan and having faith that the plan will unfold because you are you. And you are quietly saluting your strengths each day. The determination of what you had intended means to some degree having detachment from how it will happen, and having faith that it will happen, but that within you is already begining.

BEYOND BIRTHING

The early days.

YOUR PHYSICAL BODY

Your Physical body and enjoying it's shape as postpartum form enjoying its differences. Your body will take new shape. Normalising from day one into your post partum body. Love every lumpy, wobbly, stretched, gorgeousness of the expansion that has been.

Embrace every line, every change in your silhouette and look at your baby and see what you did there.

 Have a loose image of how you want your body to work into through the coming months. Make a plan and then stick to it.

Some times we benefit from the emotional kick up the arse of "oh my god I have to". This is not the time to experience that. Be kind, compassionate and take small steps each day. Observe your body. At this point you are playing the long game. Rome was built through time so, every day you do something, every day some sort of activity some sort of purposeful intended act. A workout, a long stroll with the buggy, a salad, and then another, and another and another. Remember with body it is the long game. "Consistency builds momentum and in life momentum wins " Joe de Sena . It's not the size of the act but the sequence and assimilation of the number of acts in sequence forming a new path. The say great amounts of money can be formed from the accumulation of small sums. If you imagine a river starts as a droplet, after droplet forging a path in the earth, and with each droplet becomes stronger and stronger forming a path a strong flowing a river.

Being gentle with your expectations as you would be for baby in its development. Having a sense of compassion that you would afford others towards you. You can expect a dip. postpartum. Chemically. It's natural, the importance is you do not get lost in this. Expect it and plan for it. Because then it will not creep to you and take you unawares. It isn't just you are ok and there is hope. It will pass. You are a good mum, you are still learning still bonding with baby and still beginning to appreciate. Being aware that it will happen makes it easier.

Be very present in your body. Enjoy some trees a green open space, the woods the ocean to a place of nature. And notice how your perception changes and how the space between you and them is a very different resonance. Move your body and detach in some way to a different purpose and the tension between you and baby will dissolve. It's often that you so desperately want them to sleep, for you own motive, yet they want to sleep too, and the interplay is likely the thing that is preventing either. So take a breath. One thing to embrace and embody at these moments. " It is only a matter of time " when you are desperate to sleep or finish the feed, because you are so tired. It's is only a matter of time before their eyes close and they sleep. It's is only a matter of time before they finish the feed it is only a matter of time. Say this to yourself.

It will become one of the most calming and grounding sentences in your vocabulary. And a very powerful mantra. Just like with everything. It is only a matter of time.

There is a point in Setting intention for you. Each of the areas of your life Family Work career / change continue This is where you can dream these plans as part of your self care routine. Part of your routine. As your mainstay your central focus for some people it is their romantic partner/ others it's a life they have envisaged. The questions so many people ask but do not realise is so simple. centring your heart. When your mind and heart are in alignment there is very clear intentions. It is either a yes or a no.

POST PARTUM PROMISE

your promise to you - pre loaded

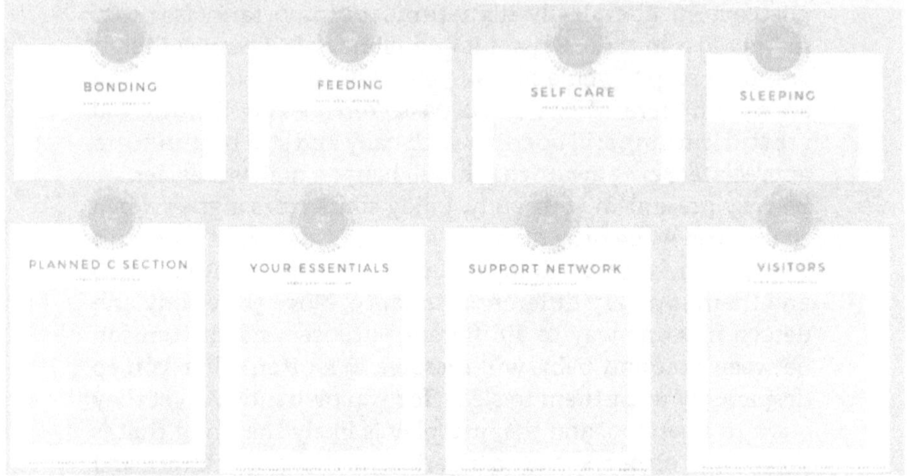

Some people consider their family on some level a drain, a drag, a weight. One of the greatest assets and grounding alignment is the love you have for you and your family. It's instinctive. They make you and never break you. That is certain. When your belief is this way you always have a strength. When you are tired it wanes. That's why you nourish.

When the inner strength you have will always be aligned with you as a mother to your children and the life you envisaged for them. They become a guiding force now, in every choice you make. It is daunting but in time it becomes you to the point that you can not remember any different. Your journey changed. Without compromise. That becomes you in the heart mind alignment. It's where you determine what will become. Inclusively a mother, a woman, a lover, a partner, a professional and a parent to your children. It will become something of greater strength to prioritise yourself as a mother and your central recovery sustenance nourishment rejuvenation will return your children make you younger as they grow older. Your children bring life to you, through you. Your children are always an asset, they become the centre within your life from birth forwards. When you see it this way, even if you miss out on the parties, the late nights the things you " used to " do. The time and attention you used to do that with has new purpose.

Being a parent will challenge you in ways unknown Children will challenge you, that is all part of the joy.

You guide them with your love. You can't feel love when you are missing the parties. You get excited about the things you love about being a parent. That's the new level for the playing field. Which is how the core alignment works effectively. You can move forward from any situation because you have the central heart alignment which will always call you to you. That is the difference in the perseverance, you have that is to be called and to be known and accepted. It isn't even a conscious concept because the heart does not speak, It moves you, it moves you and moves things and it makes some of the greatest calls of all without us even knowing, so look after it. There is a book by Greg Braden called the Divine Matrix. The most moving essence for me and my understanding of life, love and the matrix of energy in life was that envisioning. Believing are enough to make your world change to move your world in the direction of your desire, but also when you resonate with your most divine heart that is one beyond the words you know. See it believe it and then feel it as if it can come to fruition. But the real real love comes from real faith. The one that spans oceans and mountains and galaxies to bring you what you want from the great beyond. It's a sense and power that becomes you in the movements when you have almost a primal call within you for something to change, to make or to do. For peace. For surrender for support for something that you crave. This is the heart mind alignment when your hearts greatest wishes will become to life, when you centre and come one with your heart. Relax and visualise the very things you aspire to attain when you have a tiny window of time in your day. You have one heart one mind. And they both know the answer. To move forward into the solution. You have a commitment to receiving.

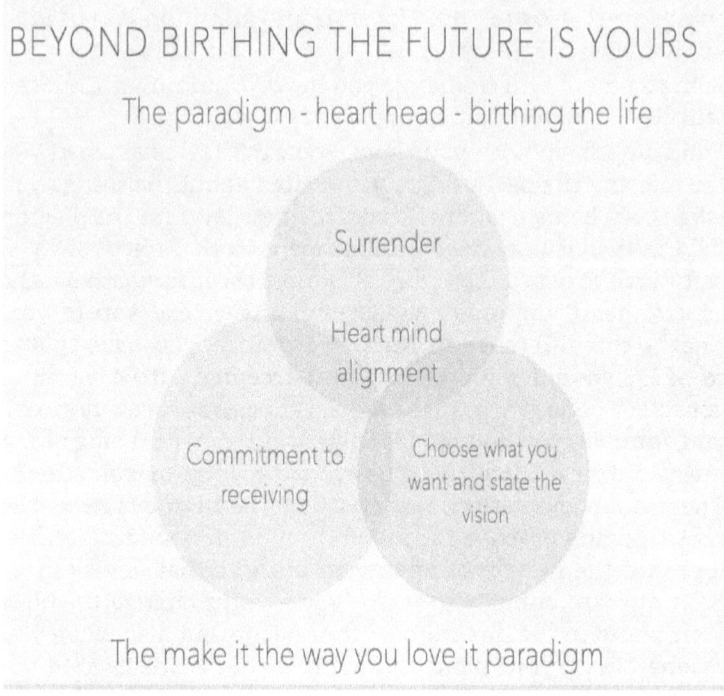

So what is next... Imagining, Envisioning the what you love.

Being mindful, centred alert to the now. Mindful used to confuse me, it meant full mind. Full mind of what you are doing, being, experiencing. Attentive to fill your attention span with what it is that you are doing and the fullest of intention of the here and now, not what upset you, or what you have got to do next, but the moment and movement you are in. We ignore the moment and get lost in the doing. Doing with intention. Living with intention. So many times we are on auto pilot. Which is an asset auto pilot with direction and alignment is more fulfilling in to life though. Always have something to move towards always have something to move into that cements you into your vision for life. To live the vision and envision. For me at one time it was the label of a swimsuit. Deep in lock down in 2020. I had a swimsuit. I think it cost £125. From a cornish founded company, a Registered B corp. They make some very beautiful clothes, using recycled plastics, and are very evolutionary. It embodied almost everything that I loved in some metaphorical way. It was symbolic. I would never have known this one swimsuit and everything it is, would afford me, would carry me though the next phase of life. Hold me together and be a rock. When no-one else was there. It was recycled plastic, Navy Blue, with a cross back, Full length size 10 from the "True north" Range. It's stunning. It's shape was so perfect. I have swam in the ocean for several years. But the suit, It gave me courage. Even now people compliment me on this full-length swim suit (it is beautiful) There were days when it meant nothing to me, I was on autopilot, between places and people in greater need. And that's when I knew I had gone. I was forgotten and everything else was so loud, that I wasn't even listening. I couldn't see me, as everyone else was too loud. I was drowning in the noise of everything else. Even when the world was closed and there was no one. So I swam and I ran. In the ice cold ocean. There is no room for distraction because it is you the ocean and your survival. Everything comes back into a trajectory that aligned me. Pulled everything together, because even though it didn't feel like it, at that time. The world was still spinning, moving, time doesn't stand still even in the sense of timelessness, but it was spinning around me. When you centre, it begins to spin with you, and within you, as well as around you. Motive, and movement. Something so small can be a huge symbol. Of faith. Courage and determination. To move forwards. Even in the darkest most solitary of times. One human just like many of you, working front line with covid patients, taking care of my parents from distance, home working, maintaining and building a business, home schooling two children. Lone parenting. The swimsuit and the ice cold water was my rock.

So no matter how tired you become, no matter the challenge you are still so much more than you imagine. But, it is so important to find your mainstay. And use it.

When your only accountability is you. What is your reminder. There is a place where you can go to make these acknowledgements to you. Where you return to yourself. Because when it is your life, your change. You set the bar.

Barriers

Time : The greatest excuse most people have is that they don't have time. Even when they don't have a new born baby in their arms. It is the greatest asset you have. The truth is. We all have 24 hour days its just a case of how you choose to spend your time. You will learn over the next few months you can survive and even thrive on regular 5 hour sleep nights /

days. You will wake with a hunger and you will enjoy your time. Because you plan to. You have motive and you have determination to make the time you have work for you then the way you live time is different. The way you live becomes more present and you get more done. Because you have direction. Heart mind alignment is about centeredness and regaining the control of your internal compass. You can do this even with a new-born. We all have 24 hour days. Within that space there is ultimate potential to make room for the enjoyment and evolution of many things. Time is precious.

Repeated small acts consistently have greater momentum. Daily acts. Which you can do even if you have a young baby. Find pockets of time to be dedicated to you. We all have the ability to visualise. We all have the ability to change our circumstances, not just out of what we don't want, but refinement. When we focus enough. For example. It's possible to make anything. I made a house, with the level of detail to the door handles. Within about 6 months with grace I did not own that one which was the intention. The next house I made was there in just 6 weeks, even with a 6 month old baby and a three year old. Just by intending to move home and saying to myself what view would I like from the window (as I was looking at a slaughter house at the bottom of the small garden.) and I said. Project green fields. This home has ocean views and fields to three sides. Panoramic Ocean views from all bedrooms, and is literally at the edge of the earth two fields from the south west coast path in a small but beautiful small village. 10 minutes walk from the beach. It can be anything you want. You see your mind is always absorbing, when you see things you like make note, they are listed and will form part of what you make. The things you really really desire. Invisibly they will list and when you vision board it becomes stronger. Your ability to visualise is always there when you are feeding baby. When you are hanging the washing out when you are cleaning when you are going about your daily chores and when you are doing just about anything. You are able to visualise with the intentions of your heart mind alignment. With simple practice of even vision boarding so the reminder is there daily every day when you forget. You have but three steps. The make it the way you love it paradigm. Choose what you want and state the vision Heart mind alignment confirm and if there is any wavering get clear in what you want. Surrender. Commitment to receiving.

Being willing to Change and having the perseverance to continue. The mental and physical strength and commitment to continue, which is why it is so important to look after your physical body and eat good food. It also gives your body and mind the impression that quality is important. Food which is healthy and nourish your mind with informational sources which inspire you. Which encourage you to be more, and to stay centred in your physical body. That will enable you to become more stable as per the earlier diagrams so you can sustain your life, and grow. Move with assertion in each and every single act. Move with intention, as you do you will be aware of your body, your health, and aware of what you are doing. It's easy to move with autopilot, but the more you move your consciousness with intention and consciously move, the more your life will continue to pull together and support you moving forwards. If you believe you can it will happen. Most of all. The more you believe you build the hue the bullet proof shield which becomes impermeable to the doubts and you can indeed succeed. The more congruent you are the more quickly it will happen. You have to have faith and certainty that some thing good will happen. Even when it does not appear so you have an unwavering faith in that what you intend will happen and is happening for you to experience at some point in time. Even if you can't see it. Trusting everything you are doing in this moment is aligned with my intentions for a fulfilling life. When you set your intentions previous to now you made a path of intention. This is amplified the more you envision it. Being open to receiving means being accepting that you are deserving of what you had intended. Give yourself permission to have it.

Surrender, how do you surrender when it is something you want fervently. When you want it so badly that you could burst. You just see it think it, believe it love it and surrender. You surrender. Being always willing to let it go. The sense that if it is right for you it will be for you. But with the determination to let nothing stand in your way. Much like balancing the science and the nature of birthing babies. Surrender what is and what is right will come to you. Like the door handles. It is accelerated. Especially when you release negative emotions and fears as you have through this evolutionary text. This includes all areas of your life, short term long term. All of the terms. You can easily do this, make a list vison board it and then allow yourself the opportunity to make it so. Give your self permission. Give yourself permission to live. Give yourself permission to be. Give your self permission to not just live, but to flourish. And then do it again , and again, and again, and again... and never stop. So there you are. You Have it. You have the keys to birthing baby. With calm confidence, ease and grace.

You can recap so now you are pregnant. You know why, You definitely know how, and you have an understanding how hypnosis for child birth works, you have experienced it. You know about your body, it makes sense now, that relaxation isn't a huge ask at all, youre aware of the influence of your hormones and know how to work your nervous system in your favour at all times. Also The Love drug oxytocin is your best friend. And so are the ways to make it.... You know the science of fear, how to reduce it, You have the mental ways the physical ways and the environmental ways. You know how to influence your hormone balance and reduce stress hormones to the positive for the purpose you have for birthing babies. you know how to breathe, you know how to You have overcome many fears, and turned them into confidences. You know how to breathe, forever to bring you calm. You have a confidence prelude to a c sections even if it is unplanned. You know how to increase your pain tolerance, to reduce discomfort. You know about mediation, you know you can make choices, and you know when labour is here what to do. You know how to mould your thoughts by using positive affirmations. You know how to communicate and encourage your partner to embrace your relationship and birth baby together as a team. You have ideas of positioning for ease. You have the ability to increase your comfort just by moving your body. You have the ability to Breathe and maintain your energy to enhance the stability of your energy and nourish your body and your mind to consistently fulfil your physical desires and to be an excellent well nourished inspired and uplifted mother and parent. You have the ability to foresee and to envision the life you want. The life to be lived, and to make the very best life for yourself an your family. You have access to the audio sessions for a nominal fee. And you know It is more than hypnobirthing it is establishing a new way of living and thinking as you move forward into parent hood. We all want the best for our children we all aspire to be the best parents we can be and we all have aspirations for our lives as parents moving forward and for our children so this is the

HOW to set about the ripple in your mind, the ripple in your life that is going to make that happen. You can't not say that now you know how. Listen, read, learn, change and then allow the unfolding of life allow the unfolding of you and unfolding of life beyond birth. So now birth, and live forward very gently but certainly empowered.

"You are my sun, my moon, and all of my stars." — E.E. Cummings

1. Teacher: "Give me a sentence about a public servant."
Student: "The fireman came down the ladder pregnant." Teacher: "Do you know what pregnant means?" Student: "Yes, it means you're carrying a child."

Quote - scarymommy.com

◆ ◆ ◆

Cesearean rehearsal

Simply close you eyes and let everything else fade away in importance

I want you to think of the word relax ……

Think about how it has two syllables

Relax…

As you breathe in think

Re to yourself

And as you breathe out

Think lax

Don't let your mind wander away for repeating the word relax

When you breathe out try to let go of any tension in your body

Focus on those muscles, which may have been holding some tension

Every tie you breathe out lax the out breath is the one to focus on

The in breath takes care of itself

Think re on each breath in and lax on each breath out

Imagine those out breaths Are being blown into a big balloon all of your tensions being expelled from your body and being blown into that big balloon The balloon being filled up with air and when it is full imagine it floating away And as it floats away the balloon carries away all of those tensions And you Reeel aaaax You reee laaaax Calm confident and in control Each breath And you are feeling completely in control Allow your hands to rest comfortably on top of your legs wherever they feel most comfortable Now as you relax more and let it go ore and more You can allow every muscle in your body to relax Every cell every nerve every fiber in your body relaxing Now picture in your mind a candle this candle can be any color you with it to be The color you have chose n for your candle is a color you unconscious mind knows relaxes you and calms your mind Calms you and relaxes your mind. It is your color of calm Now focus on you the color of the flame of the candle See how amazing the colors within the flame are You may see red, blue yellow purple white And maybe another color And as you see the colors within the flame you relax more and more And go deeper And as you enjoy these heavy and relaxed feelings deeply relaxed feelings These feelings of being in control. Now focus on the wax body of your candle Now see the first trickle of melting wax begin to move down the wax Now see the melting wax touch the candleholder and merge with it to become part of the candleholder You become more and more relaxed Feeling safe and comfortable Now imagine that you re that candle A candle of total relaxation Now within this relaxation you can think towards a safe place inside Within that safe place you will have a space to build ne experience of the unknown. You can imagine now that you are within the preparation for your theatre you are prepared and feeling calm confident and in control your re surrounded by professionals who know what to do to help you birth your baby So you can be calm confident and in control The room smells clinical and that's of comfort, as you know it's a safe way to right baby on this day The sounds the colors you can acclimatize very quickly

You remember the candle the candle of ultimate relaxation Any nerves or fears can simply dissolve as you have a sense of comfort and priority to bright baby with ease faith love ad safely maintaining that sense of comfort always knowing that you are doing the right thing for you and the right thing for baby And you remember the candle the candle of ultimate relaxation and feel calm confident and in control The sense of the room is professional and clean though you have the sense of growing warmth and love within you building and building and feeling of greater comfort You move towards the theater and as you go rethought doors you can small the clean and fresh environment you can sense the setting is ok, it is safe and you feel comfortable to proceed with the procedure As you prepare you may be required to lie down or sit upon the edge of the bed for a small numbing treatment. It feels totally normal. It feels totally comfortable. You know what to expect. You are calm confident and in control any fears or worries can just release as you breathe in calm and breathe out tension breathe in calm and breathe out tension As you do you feel calm confident and strong within Each moment is taking you closer to birthing your baby safely Each and every breath you take is bringing you closer to birthing your baby so you enter into the theatre and you lie on the table The clothes and gowns and masks feel appropriate and you have a growing sense of comfort knowing that each moment is bringing you closer to birthing your baby You can hear the instruments whirring in the background and the light are bright and that feels comfortable You have a sense of warmth and comfort within you through you and around you and a strong sense also to enjoy the experience of birthing baby To be aware and to be alive and to feel the comfortable sense of calm confident awareness growing within you As you look up and see the gowns and the doctors at their work you may hear the tinkling of the medical instruments in the room and each moment and each sound that you recognize gives you a deepening sense of comfort and sense of control within that comfort knowing that each breath and each moment that passes is bringing you closer to birthing your baby As time passes the surgeons may speak with you and update you they will guide you so you know what is happening movement by movement And the sense of comfort within you remains strong with each breath in As you take one now and relax knowing that everything is ok And you remember the candle the candle of ultimate relaxation and feel calm confident and in control As you hear the sound of the tinkling instruments and you may feel sense of pressure under your ribs just before baby is born As you do you breathe in and relax and allow the process to continue knowing that each moment and each breath brings you closer to birthing your baby Any discomfort you can remember the candle within and the dials the internal dials to switch down the discomfort once its message has been heard you can turn the dials down Then you can hear the sound of your baby's cry as you imagine looking up and baby is there. So your body can now begin to synthesize the hormone oxytocin the love drug because it can and it can increase the sense of love and healing for your body and for bonding with t baby. The moment you hear baby's cry's and see baby your body responds t the birth with the production of the love hormone so you can accelerate your physical healing and form bond with baby and move through the coming hours days and weeks with a strong sense of love bonding with baby feeding baby and bonding with baby And you remember the candle the candle of ultimate relaxation and feel calm confident and in control as you see the candle in your minds eye you know your body is healing and using it energy and nutrients to birth you and baby Your body can heal and is healing every breath you now take without conscious the ought or effort you are now healing while loving baby Bond with a baby and feel baby on your skin your body's natural response immediately as baby bonds with you bond with baby and feel that deepening sense of strength and comfort as you progress the sense of comfort you have is deepening and beginning fill your whole body that sense of great love and joy combined as the relief that baby is here There resting on your chest You can smell them and feel their tiny arms and legs moving now outside of your body and the beauty of the experience is all encompassing The love with you and baby and that moment will be within you for the whole of your life together and always be safe and protected in your mind and remembered when needed so you can stay calm confident and in control if you ever experience a sense of unease or not enough ness you can remember that bond that strength that love and that love will move you forward to make the very best things happen . And you take a deep breath in and this memory begins to fade but it fades into moments and seconds of your future time and living memory so it becomes to the future so you can stay firmly present in the now and enjoy each moment of pregnancy throughout. And as you do you can remaining very relaxed take a few moments to breathe in and out and in And out and then as I count form one to 10 on the number ten you will awaken alert and in the room.

One

Two

Three

Four

Five

Six

Seven

Eight

Nine

Ten

All content and images © Victoria Whitney 2024

◆ ◆ ◆

[1] Wikipedia - https://en.wikipedia.org/wiki/Franz_Mesmer
[2] https://www.hopkinsmedicine.org/health/conditions-and-diseases/staying-healthy-during-pregnancy/4-common-pregnancy-complications
[3] https://www.ncbi.nlm.nih.gov/pmc/articles/PMC7120324/
[4] https://pubmed.ncbi.nlm.nih.gov/21762655/

[5] https://www.ncbi.nlm.nih.gov/pmc/articles/PMC9136365/

[6] https://victoria-s-school-f8ca.thinkific.com/

[7] http://victoriawhitney.com/ - online courses tab.

____

[i] https://abcnews.go.com/Health/story?id=117313&page=1
https://www.indiatoday.in/india/story/woman-in-coma-for-7-months-gives-birth-to-baby-girl-at-delhi-aiims-2291104-2022-10-30
https://www.deccanherald.com/content/183487/british-woman-gives-birth-coma.html

AFTERWORD

The materials in Victoria Whitney's books are provided on an as is basis.

For the purposes of education and entertainment. Victoria Whitney makes no warranties expressed or implied and hereby disclaims and negates all other warranties included within content, online courses trainings, including without limitation. Implied warranties or conditions of merchantability fitness for a particular purpose or non infringement of intellectual property, contestation of service delivery as described or other violation of rights.

Further Victoria Whitney does not warrant or make any representation concerning the accuracy likely of results or reliability of the use of terms on consultation or materials on its books or programs of guidance used in sessions and recommended or otherwise such relating to the to the materials on this site and session content.

The information in this book is based on the author's knowledge, experience and opinions. The methods described in this book are not intended to be a definitive set of instructions. You may discover other methods and materials to accomplish the same end result. Your results may differ.

There are no representations or warranties, express or implied, about the completeness, accuracy, or reliability of the information, products, services, or related materials contained in this book. The information is provided "as is," to be used entirely at your own risk.

This book is not intended to give legal or financial advice and is sold with the understanding that the author is not engaged in rendering legal, accounting or other professional services or advice. If legal or financial advice or other expert assistance is required, the services of a competent professional should be sought to ensure you fully understand your obligations and risks.

This book includes information regarding the products and services of third parties. We do not assume responsibility for any third party materials or opinions. Use of mentioned third party materials does not guarantee your results will mirror those mentioned in the book.

All trademarks appearing in this book are the property of their respective owners.

This book may not be re-sold or given away to other people. If you like to share this book with another person, please purchase an additional copy for each person you share it with.

The publisher and the author strongly recommend that you consult with your physician before beginning any exercise program. You should be in good physical condition and be able to participate in the exercises expressed within this book. The author is not a licensed healthcare care provider and represents that they have no expertise in diagnosing, examining, or treating medical conditions of any kind, or in determining the effect of any specific exercise on a medical condition.

You should understand that at any time during labour you could require the assistance of medical professional.

Always seek medical advice if you are concerned. The author and publisher accepts no responsibility or liability for failure to do so. OR any representative damage, personal physical or otherwise, or loss which could occur as a result from the omission to do so.

If you engage in these activities Scripts and guidance does not replace the requirement for professional medical advice. IN reading this book and using these practices you, you agree that you do so at your own risk, are voluntarily participating in these activities, assume all risk of injury to yourself, and agree to release and discharge the publisher and the author from any and all claims or causes of action, known or unknown, arising out of the contents of this book.

The publisher and the author advise you to take full responsibility for your safety and know your limits. Before practicing the skills described in this book, be sure that your equipment is well maintained and do not take risks beyond your level of experience, aptitude, training, Condition of health and mind and comfort level.

Although the publisher and the author have made every effort to ensure that the information in this book was correct at press time and while this publication is designed to provide accurate information in regard to the subject matter covered, the publisher and the author assume no responsibility for errors, inaccuracies, omissions, or any other inconsistencies herein and hereby disclaim any liability to any party for any loss, damage, or disruption caused by errors or omissions, whether such errors or omissions result from negligence, accident, or any other cause.

Unless otherwise indicated, all the names, characters, businesses, places, events and incidents in this book are either the product of the author's imagination or used in a fictitious manner. Any resemblance to actual persons, living or dead, or actual events is purely coincidental.

The publisher and the author make no guarantees concerning the level of success you may experience by following the advice and strategies contained in this book, and you accept the risk that results will differ for each individual. The testimonials and examples provided in this book show exceptional results, which may not apply to the average reader, and are not intended to represent or guarantee that you will achieve the same or similar results.

This book is not intended as a substitute for the medical advice of physicians. The reader should regularly consult a physician in matters relating to their health, particularly with respect to any symptoms that may require diagnosis or medical attention.

ACKNOWLEDGEMENT

The contents of this book are advisory capacity only You should always check with a medical doctor before undertaking any new routine relative to health especially during pregnancy.

Victoria and Birthing babies accepts no liability for actions taken and choices made as a result of reading and using any of the materials included in this book. Medical guidance is always advised without question through out your pregnancy, and birth.

 This book is for personal private or non commercial use

This is grant of a license not a transfer of a title.
All content and images Copyright Victoria Whitney © 2024

Victoria Disclaims liability for damages or loss of data, personal gain or profit or due to business interruption arising out of the use or inability to use the materials on Victoria Whitney's book, video or audio recordings directly or linked to third party sites or distributed for your own personal and private use by Victoria Whitney or third parties eg thinkific, Amazon.

5. Accuracy of materials

These materials appearing within this text could include technical typographical or photographic content or errors

Victoria Whitney does not warrant that any of the materials on this book are accurate complete or current though makes best efforts to ensure they are so. Victoria Whitney may make changes to these materials contained on its book and re publish at any time without notice however Victoria does not make any commitment to update materials.

6. links

Victoria Whitney has not reviewed all of the sites linked to its book and is not responsible for the contents of any such linked site The inclusion of any link does not imply endorsement by Victoria Whitney of this site use of any such linked website is at the owners risk

7. Health and contraindications – Victoria disclaims liability and gives express advice to consult a medical doctor if you have any underlying health condition. Known or unknown before using any of the practices in this book.

ABOUT THE AUTHOR

Victoria Whitney

welcome to "birthing babies" The aim.
To make Hypnotherpay for child birth a simple as possible as accessible as possible and enable women to have an empowered birth.
To build calm, clarity and confidence in women who birth. so they can feel empowered in their own bodies to birth their babies.
Victoria Whitney is an Award Winning Personal Empowerment Expert. mum. Ultra marathon runner. Ocean lover. She have birthed two babies and empowered many women in life with World class change techniques as a profession and to birth their babies with confidence using hypnotherapy for child birth.
She been a Coach and trainer of Hypnotherapy for 15 years, hypnotic birthing process practitioner for the last 10 years and have blended these loves and her experience and knowledge of birthing mindset and the mind body connection to form this course so you can be empowered to birth your baby calmly and confidently and flow on your journey form birth to motherhood.